Hormones Explained

Hormones Explained

Anti-aging Medicine,
Bioidentical Hormone Replacement Therapy,
and the Controversies

Dr. Selma Rashid, M.D.

www.hormonesexplained.com

Order this book online at:
www.hormonesexplained.com

Printed in Great Britain.

ISBN: 978-1-4507-1015-2

CHAPELPRESS   Printed by Chapel Press

Contents

Chapter 18
Treatment with Ovarian Hormones (Estrogen and Progesterone) 95

Chapter 19
Testosterone in Women 104

Chapter 20
Testosterone Replacement in Men 107

Chapter 1

Introduction

"I will prevent disease whenever I can, for prevention is preferable to cure"
"I will apply, for the benefit of the sick, all measures [that] are required,
avoiding those twin traps of overtreatment and therapeutic nihilism."
(From the Hippocratic Oath: Modern Version)

A Dysfunctional Medical System

In many countries, somewhere along the way, healthcare lost track of its responsibilities and became a business. As a result, aging people in many developed nations are more medicated and unhealthier than ever before, while giant organizations such as the pharmaceutical industry have evolved even further, exploiting the name of medicine for massive profits. It is in such countries that the oath of medicine has been dishonored, and the medical industry is doing more harm than good, without the best possible options being offered.

The U.S. healthcare system in particular has become a prime example of medical mismanagement, spending the most on healthcare than any other nation yet ranking below twentieth in quality of health. Until consumers understand what is going on around them, they will continue to be targets of a system adulterated by corruption and ignorance.

Very simply, if a medical treatment makes money and is patentable, it becomes first in line for approval and part of standard medicine. If it is not patentable and cuts into the profits of the present system, it is usually dishonored and kept out of the mainstream.

Health—Our Greatest Asset and Our Greatest Fear

The most valuable asset we have is our health, and one of our greatest fears is losing our functionality. No wealth in the world can calm the anguish of a disabling stroke, and there are very few diagnoses that have the impact as the soul-shaking diagnosis of cancer. We fear Alzheimer's disease, which may cause such severe mental deterioration that we might not recognize our own children. Yet, we continue to put our trust in the hands of the medical system hoping they have our best interests at heart.

Exploring the Truth

Hormonal balance is crucial to health and functionality. Fortunately, throughout the world, many brilliant scientist and physicians are pursuing advanced medical concepts that will help us to understand the diseases of aging, as well as the significance of hormone balance We are realizing that everything we are exposed to affects our wellbeing. With a healthy body and environment, the correct replacement of diminishing hormones can significantly eliminate the diseases of aging.

Individuals as well as the economy benefit from health and functionality. Waiting for the signs and symptoms of disease rather than working to prevent them is a losing battle and a financial burden; taking the correct measures at the right time is more feasible and financially manageable.

Chapter 2

Aging and Disease

Onset of Aging

As we age, most of us are not tuned to respond to the onset of the aging process. We are embarrassed to acknowledge our signs of aging and are discouraged to discuss them until they become a classic disease.

There are many symptoms that signify the onset of aging. For example, the body's metabolic rate slows down, and losing weight becomes more difficult. We have less energy, are more tired, have increased body pain, and diminished sexual function, among other symptoms. These symptoms usually start in the fourth and fifth decades of life.

Early intervention, with advanced preventive measures, can help us avoid the deterioration of our health and prevent the diseases to which we are genetically predisposed.

Some common age-related diseases are:
- Type 11 diabetes
- Stroke
- Hypertension
- Dyslipidemia
- Alzheimer's disease
- Parkinson's disease
- Cardiovascular disease
- Arthritis
- Osteoporosis
- Chronic fatigue and fibromyalgia
- Autoimmune diseases
- Digestive system disorders

- Age related cancers
- Depression and mood disorders
- Memory loss
- Sexual dysfunction

Age-related diseases do not begin overnight. The disease process starts many years before the first signs appear. Certain age-related diseases have a genetic predisposition, while others are influenced by lifestyle and the environment.

Management of Health in the Elderly

The quality of health and medical management of the elderly is disturbingly poor. Most of the elderly in advanced nations are overmedicated and debilitated with the side effects, without any significant increase in their quality of health.

Spending our later lives in a nursing home is an unpleasant thought, a situation almost everyone wants to avoid. Nursing home residents were asked which of their medical problems disturbed them the most. Pain—usually from arthritis—was the most common response. Those who had lost function from stroke wanted to be able to walk and use the bathroom without calling for help. Many wished they had more energy and did not feel constantly tired. Almost all felt they were a burden and felt pride in remembering their days of health.

Americans are the only people in the world who readily take prescription medications without much question, blindly trusting what their physicians and the pharmaceutical industry are providing. People in other countries have access to the same drugs used in the United States, at much less cost, but they are far more discerning about using them.

Trends in Healthcare

The most dramatic changes in medicine occurred in the last century with the introduction of antibiotics, anesthesia, vaccinations, and antiseptics. These advancements increased the average age of survival from the late forties to the early eighties, but provided no increase in the quality of health.

The Start of the Medical Business

The increase in the aging population has enabled medicine to become a booming business, with hospitals, pharmaceutical companies, medical device companies, and nursing homes earning record profits and convincing us that we are receiving the best medical care in the world.

The *Canadian Medical Association Journal* published an article in which researchers sought to evaluate the prediction that from 2000 to 2025 there will be a 24 percent increase in the incidence of hypertension in developed countries. Their results showed that this is an underestimation, and that the actual rise will likely far exceed the predicted numbers.[1]

U.S. government Centers for Disease Control (CDC) records show that adult onset diabetes is increasing[2] and other records show that antidepressants have become the most commonly prescribed class of medications in the United States.[3]

Preparing for More Success

The baby boomers, now entering their "aging years," will undoubtedly suffer from a multitude of age-related diseases. The statistics projected for the increase in age-related diseases has triggered a nationwide growth in the number of hospitals. The number of physicians specializing in hospital medicine—and the demand for them—is increasing.[4, 5]

There is no plan in sight for disease prevention. The urgency appears to be only in treatment. The U.S. healthcare system is sustained by the presence of disease. Without disease, there is minimal requirement for pharmaceutical drugs, hospitalization, and nursing homes.

Chapter 3

Different Approaches to Health Management

The Advanced Medical Approach to Aging

Physicians across the world have taken an active role in understanding the disease process and the aging process from the foundations of medical science, with the goal of preventing age-related diseases and maintaining functionality. This field of medicine is generally referred to as anti-aging medicine and has made remarkable progress; however, it presently lacks standardization.

Some general principles of the advanced medical approach are:

- Preventative measures can be developed if we can understand the process of disease.
- The earlier the body is brought back to balance when symptoms occur, the less likely it is that the symptoms will progress to disease and dysfunction.
- Pharmaceutical drugs and surgeries have an important role in medicine, but should not be used for routine medical management.
- Elderly patients benefit greatly by emphasis on correct nutritional support, replacement of diminished hormones, and minimal use of pharmaceutical drugs.
- Human bodies are designed to recognize imbalance. Most people become frustrated when their state of well-being starts to decline, but are reluctant to take action due to lack of knowledge and direction.
- Taking timely corrective measures results in optimal health.

The Traditional Medical Approach—"Standard of Care"

The traditional medical approach, also known as standard-of-care medicine, does not focus on prevention, but does make money on age-related diseases:

- Traditional medicine follows strict guidelines set forth by the nation's board of medicine in each specialty including surgery.

- Traditional medicine deals with classic diseases, which can be treated surgically or pharmaceutically. However, it does not address the prevention of age-related diseases in any significant manner.

- Treating age-related diseases is lucrative for the present medical system but disabling and expensive for the consumer.

- Many of the treatments in traditional, standard-of-care medicine are invaluable and have no substitute. However, if age-related diseases were eliminated, so would the bulk of the business for the present health system.

Alternative and Integrative Medicine

Alternative medicine generally involves health providers who use non-pharmaceutical and non-surgical methods to address disease. Although many of these methods are useful, they are not backed with the level of research, regulation, or standardization as methods used by traditional medicine.

The field of integrative medicine combines traditional medical approaches with alternative medicine. Although these methods have proven beneficial in many cases, they too are backed by limited standardization and regulation.

Integrative and alternative medicine, like traditional, standard-of-care medicine, treat diseases and have negligible focus on the prevention of age-related diseases.

The Medical Goal

The goal of medicine should be the complete prevention of all age-related diseases. The medical literature is full of scientific studies and data on how the disease process starts and progresses. If this information could be developed, aging could be a graceful and enjoyable experience.

Chapter 4

Example of Medical Mismanagement of an Age-Related Disease

Cardiovascular disease has been the leading cause of death over the last several decades. The disease results in the tragic consequences of stroke, heart attack, and death. The annual cost for treating heart disease was $60 billion in 1991,[6] the cost now is far greater.

High blood pressure and elevated cholesterol are two major contributing factors to heart disease. Both of these conditions could be could be avoided if managed correctly. For example:

High Blood Pressure (Hypertension)

High blood pressure is one of the leading causes of death in the modern world. The process starts several years before the numbers cause concern.

It has also been medically recognized that, when women lose their hormonal protection at menopause, their rate of heart disease rapidly increases.[7]

Steps leading to high blood pressure (simplified):

- The body's metabolic system slows down, and cell function declines. Effective repair of routine cell damage cannot occur.

- During the same time, calcium balance is compromised. Rather than going back into the bone, calcium starts to build up in blood vessel walls, making them stiff. Calcium is also lost through urine. As expected, this is also the time osteoporosis begins.

- Loss of elasticity in the blood vessel walls with the addition of calcification causes the arteries to become hardened, while veins become floppy. The declining cell function cannot repair damage as it did in earlier years.

- The combination of calcification and age-related degeneration of the blood vessel walls causes the mean blood pressure to rise. Over time, the arteries become increasingly damaged, weakened, and brittle.

- If the pressure is high enough, a weakened blood vessel may rupture. This can result in a hemorrhagic (bleeding) stroke. If there is an arterial plaque, it could be dislodged and block a smaller vessel. This can result in an ischemic (blockage type) stroke or a heart attack.

- Veins, due to a different set of mechanics and structure, become floppy with aging. The valves which prevent backflow become damaged and blood is not sent back to the heart as efficiently, leading to swelling of the lower extremities.

- When the body's fluid balance is upset, hypertension worsens in a very predictable sequence.

Traditional medicine accepts an increase in mean blood pressure as a normal aging process. After an arbitrary number for blood pressure is reached, pharmaceutical drugs are used to slow down the blood force. As the disease progresses, diuretics are given to remove swelling. In the event of a stroke or heart attack, more drugs are added. The real medical problem is never addressed, solved, or treated.

If the calcium balance can be maintained and the blood vessel walls can be kept healthy, blood pressure would not rise. This loss in the balance of health is largely due to declining cell health and diminishing hormones.

Elevated Blood Cholesterol

Elevated blood cholesterol is frustratingly mismanaged in standard medicine. To treat the problem, it first needs to be correctly understood.

- Cholesterol is a vital molecule for life. It is used by the cells to form many components essential for life, including steroid hormones, neurosteroids, vitamin D, as well as the components of cell membranes and the nervous system.

- A high blood cholesterol number indicates that cholesterol is not entering the cells, which means it is not being used.

- Because cholesterol is so critical for life, if the cells do not detect enough of it, they send a message to the liver to synthesize more. Neither the cells nor the liver seem to sense when the cholesterol is too high in the blood.

- Cholesterol travels in the body attached to certain carrier proteins, most notably low-density lipoprotein (LDL). In order for cells to be able to use LDL, the cells need to make LDL receptors (gates) for the cholesterol to enter. Without healthy cells and cell membranes, cholesterol stays in the blood and unable to enter the cells to be used.

- Cholesterol, especially in the form of LDL is sensitive to being oxidized (damaged) when it is in the blood too long. Oxidized LDL is "sticky" and likes to stick to damaged artery walls. This initiates a coating on the artery walls called plaque. This process is what has given LDL a bad name (it is known as "bad cholesterol"). LDL is actually critical for health; it just needs to get into the cell so that it doesn't remain in the blood for too long and then become damaged (oxidized).

- The cholesterol-deficient cells send messages to the liver to make more cholesterol; however, cholesterol-lowering medications (such as statins) stop the liver from producing more cholesterol.

- The problem of the underutilization of cholesterol is not solved with cholesterol-lowering medications. Although they cause less oxidized LDL to remain in the blood in the short term, the body suffers in the long term.

- Cholesterol medications also accelerate damage to the body by depleting it of necessary energy and contribute to further oxidizing (damaging) existing LDL.

- Steroid hormones such as estradiol as well as thyroid hormone are documented in the medical literature to improve the cholesterol profile. (See chapter 11, Steroid Hormones).

Chapter 5

Cells and Hormones in the Aging Process

THE CELL (simplified)

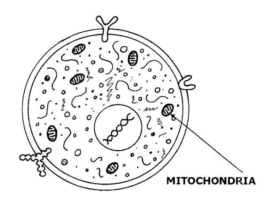

MITOCHONDRIA

The Cell

Life starts from two cells that combine and then divide into two. Each of those divides, and each subsequent cell divides. Each cell becomes specialized as it becomes part of functional tissues and organs and other necessary body parts. Throughout life, cells cycle by dividing, carrying out their functions, and dying.

During their life span, cells produce reactions and products necessary to sustain life and function. Cells are the simplest unit of life, but they function collectively. All dividing cells contain deoxyribonucleic acid (DNA), which is the genetic code that governs cell division and protein synthesis.

Cells generate energy. They produce hormones and everything else needed for life that does not come from the diet or environment.

Cell components, including the highly dynamic and complex cell membrane, need to be healthy. They need to sustain minimal metabolic and environmental damage.

Hormone Actions on the Cell

Hormones are potent chemical signals that are produced in specialized cells. Using a complex communication network, they conduct the smooth running of the body, telling the cells what to do, what to produce, and what to break down.

Hormones act on either the cells that make them, cells in close vicinity, or on cells in far-off parts of the body.

If cells are damaged or unhealthy, they become deficient in energy and unable to respond well to the hormone signals or produce adequate hormones. If the cells are otherwise healthy but hormone deficient, the body begins to deteriorate in function.

Chapter 6

Hormones

The human body cannot function without hormones, and there is no doubt that hormones need to be in balance.

Every part of the brain and body, including the different organ systems, hormones, and other chemicals work together. Nothing in the body works in isolation, and balance is critical to well-being.

We are only just beginning to understand how complex the hormone system really is. The intricate ways in which hormones communicate with each other as well as with the many other chemicals in the brain, the body, and the environment is only partially understood.

It is imperative that, when considering hormone replacement, we maintain a conservative approach, and only work with sound scientific knowledge.

Why Hormones Became Confusing and Controversial

Over the past several years, the topic of hormones has caused a lot of controversy and confusion. This is mainly because:

- Although, the scientific evidence on the benefits of hormones is overwhelming, there are no medical protocols on hormone replacement for functionality other than treating classic diseases, short-term menopausal symptoms, and infertility, as well as addressing birth control.

- Hormone replacement became highly controversial after the Women's Health Initiative (WHI) Study, a major study funded by the National Institute of Health (NIH), was halted due to adverse outcomes. The truth about this study was never explained. Only some scattered pieces of information were released, further confusing the issue. (See Chapter 16.)

• The medical community has been inadequate in recognizing and providing the truth about synthetic hormones and bioidentical hormones (molecularly identical to those manufactured by the human body).

• The use of synthetic hormones, including birth control pills, has been allowed to go on for decades unchallenged by the standard medical community.

Different Types of Hormones

There are a few different classes of hormones based on their structure type. The main classes are:

Steroid Hormones

All steroid hormones are made from cholesterol and include estrogens, testosterone, progesterone, cortisol, aldosterone, and dehydroepiandrosterone (DHEA) among others.

Estrogen, progesterone, and testosterone are considered the hormones of fertility and are the first major hormones to decline as we age. These—especially estrogen and progesterone—are also the ones that have caused the most controversy.

A decline in the hormones of fertility is directly related to a decline in youthfulness and well-being, which eventually leads to further dysfunction and disease.

Protein or Peptide Hormones

These include insulin, growth hormone, follicle-stimulating hormone (FSH), luteinizing hormone (LH), and others. Like all hormones, these generally decline with aging but not as predictably or dramatically as steroid hormones.

Amino Acid– Derived Hormones

Hormones whose structures are derived from amino acids include thyroid hormone, melatonin, and others. When these decline or become out of balance, they too cause dysfunction and disease; however, their natural decline is steady, unlike that of steroid hormones.

Three Commonly Asked Hormone-Related Questions and Answers:

1. Should I take hormones?

Anyone whose body is functioning with suboptimal levels of hormones will eventually suffer in health. The medical literature throughout the decades and around the world has provided us with exhaustive data on the benefits of hormones. The question now is not "if" one should take them, it is "how" one should take them.

2. Are hormones safe?

Hormones are safe when they are given correctly. Incorrect hormone replacement can have detrimental effects including those listed on the package inserts of birth control pills. (See chapter 14, Birth Control Pills) Hormone replacement is not correctly understood or managed by traditional standard-of-care medicine.

- Replacement hormones should be of the exact molecular structure as the hormones naturally produced by the body.

Anything else has been shown to be harmful. (See Chapter 11, Progesterone)

- Hormones are produced in the body with a rhythm and should be replaced in as close to the natural rhythm as possible. Giving hormones outside their normal rhythm can lead to imbalance, regardless of the initial feeling of well-being.

- The route of entry is important and should be considered. For example, estrogen by mouth is documented to have adverse effects on the body. Testosterone by mouth also has significant implications, especially in regard to the liver.

- The site of hormone application makes a difference. For example, the type and thickness of fat, skin density, and quality as well as other factors affect the dynamics of hormone absorption and entry into the circulation.

- If hormones are replaced, levels should be regularly monitored.

3. *Can I age naturally without hormones?*

    One will certainly age naturally without hormone replacement. However, aging naturally also means succumbing to the genetic weaknesses that cause age-related diseases such as Alzheimer's disease, cardiovascular disease, and arthritis. Also of note is that our previous generations lived in a very different health environment than ours, and therefore their aging does not serve as an accurate model for our projected aging.

Places in the Body Where Hormones are Produced

Hormones are predominantly made in cells within specialized structures called glands; for example, ovaries, testicles, thyroid gland, adrenal glands and pineal gland.

Hormones are also made in specialized cells of other organs such as the pancreas, brain, and digestive tract.

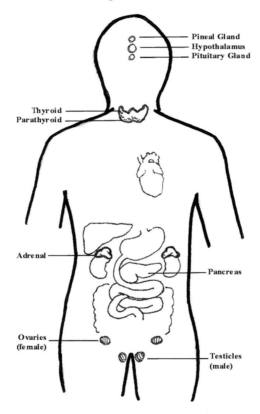

As mentioned earlier, hormones and glands do not function in isolation; rather, they closely interact with each other. The correct balance of the body's endocrine (hormone) system is essential for long-term health.

Hormone Rhythms and Patterns of Production

Every hormone is produced in a particular rhythm and interacts with other hormones and chemicals; therefore, disruption in one hormone system results in imbalances in other systems. All hormones decline in overall production through life; however, some hormones decline at a faster rate than others.

Certain hormones, such as glucagon and insulin, are produced as needed; for example, to balance blood glucose.

Other hormones, such as cortisol, melatonin, and growth hormone, are predominantly produced at specific times of the day. For example, cortisol levels should be lowest at night so we can relax and sleep, and they should be high in the morning because cortisol helps us deal with the day. On the other hand, melatonin and growth hormone work best when their levels are high at night because they work on repair and growth.

Hormone production also varies with special times of life such as during the growth and development years and during pregnancy.

Although we recognize the daily pattern for the production of some hormones, the monthly and seasonal patterns for most hormones are not yet clearly understood.

The female menstrual cycle is a unique hormone system in which estrogen and progesterone are produced in a distinct, highly regulated pattern. Many hormones do not function effectively without pulsing (in some cases at high frequency).[8] Numerous studies have demonstrated how hormones are dependent on a rhythm for optimum function.

Environmental Influences on Hormones

Over the years, common, unsuspected environmental pollutants accumulate in our bodies, especially in fat cells. These pollutants interfere with our endocrine (hormone) system.[9,10,11]

Many of the environmental pollutants contain what are known

as xenoestrogens. Xenoestrogens disrupt estrogen activity, oppose androgen (e.g., testosterone) activity, and affect thyroid function.[9,10,12,13] The extent of the human risk is still not fully known.

Many of these chemicals are passed from breast milk to infants, and many have become part of the biological food chain.[9]

The list of environmental pollutants is exhaustive and disturbing. Here are just a few examples:

- Plastics (Especially dangerous are those in which we store and heat foods and liquids. The softer the plastic, the more hazardous, because they contain more harmful additives. Water bottles are a prime example.)

- Pesticides

- Chemicals and hormone-like substances that induce faster and bigger food growth

- Lead[12]

Hormones in the Media

Hormones have been of considerable interest in the media, particularly over the past six years. This has been largely due to the controversial data on the hormones used for menopause.

Standard medical protocol has not accepted hormone replacement for functionality and disease prevention, but physicians involved in advanced preventive healthcare in the United States and internationally believe it has an important role.

Also, from time to time, we hear about athletes being apprehended for abuse of steroids that actually mimic the function of naturally produced steroid hormones.

Endocrinology

The medical subspecialty that treats hormone diseases is called endocrinology. There is no medical subspecialty that addresses prevention of disease due to inadequate hormone levels.

It is medically recognized that the endocrine system is one of the most sensitive communication networks of the human body, influencing every aspect of human well-being and health.[9]

Endocrinologists—and other medical specialists including gynecologists—are not trained in or familiar with hormone deficiencies that do not cause disease.

Birth control, menopause, and infertility are the main non-disease uses for hormones in mainstream medicine. The majority of these hormones are not real hormones, but synthetic analogs that do not exist naturally in the human body.

Anti-aging physicians who treat hormone deficiencies have no standardized method, while standard medicine does not address the issue, leaving the burden of decision on the consumer.

Summary of the Important Points about Hormones:

- Hormones serve as very potent chemical signals that intricately instruct the cells of the body how to function.

- No hormone is made in a constant, static dose but rather has a specific pattern or rhythm of production and release.

- Hormones interact with each other as well as with other potent chemicals, the brain, the entire body, and environment in intricate, complex ways that we are only beginning understand.

- After a hormone performs its function, it is broken down quickly by specific molecules called enzymes. If this does not happen, the hormone can continue to signal inappropriately.

- The major hormones are mainly produced in local structures called glands; for example, the ovaries, testes, and thyroid.

- As the body ages, it produces fewer hormones, which further slows down the cell function, and speeds the aging process.

- Replacing hormones without regard to the rhythm and dosing can lead to imbalance regardless of initial perceived benefits.

- There is ample scientific evidence that replacing diminishing hormones improves the functioning of the body;[14] however, the scientific literature does not clearly address how to replace them.

Chapter 7

Steroid Hormones

All steroid hormones are created from cholesterol. Cholesterol is one of the most misunderstood molecules in the human system, and it is imperative that we correctly understand its role in human function rather than eliminating it. The first step in steroid hormone synthesis involves cholesterol entering the mitochondia (energy-producing elements) in the cells.

Understanding Cholesterol

Cholesterol is an essential part of the human body. It is a component of countless structures in the body as well as the starting point of critical life-sustaining molecules including steroid hormones.

- Cholesterol is the normal component of cell membranes, brain tissue, and muscles as well as many other body structures.

- After birth, the body's cholesterol comes from the diet.

- In the United Kingdom, parents are cautioned to give only full-fat milk to children under three to ensure that adequate cholesterol is available for brain and nervous system development.

- Because the brain and nervous system are constantly regenerating, cholesterol continues to be a requirement throughout life.

- If the body does not have enough cholesterol to make what it needs, it will signal the liver to synthesize more.

- Without adequate cholesterol going into the cells, the body starts to decline in health and function.

- High blood cholesterol means that cholesterol is not entering the cells to be used.

- If cholesterol is not able to enter the cells and be used, the cell structures become compromised, hormonal balance is lost, and other dysfunctions are triggered.

- Eliminating cholesterol from the blood by medication is harmful in the long term. Any benefit in the short term is temporary and superficial.

- The long-term solution to balanced cholesterol is to optimize cell health, minimize oxidative damage, and balance hormones.

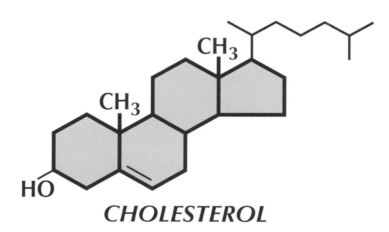

CHOLESTEROL

Steroid Hormone Synthesis

The major steroid hormones include the following:

- Progesterone
- Estrogen

- Testosterone

- Cortisol

- Aldosterone

- Dehydroepiandrosterone (DHEA)

- Androstenedione

- Pregnenolone

Steroid hormone synthesis in the human body is a complex, multistep process involving cholesterol as the starting molecule. The majority of the cholesterol needed is in the form of LDL. Every hormone-producing cell has LDL receptors (gates).

A small amount of cholesterol is also stored within the glands for immediate hormone manufacturing.

Understanding Mitochondria

The first and critical step in steroid hormone synthesis occurs in special structures in the cells called mitochondria.[15,16]

THE CELL (simplified)

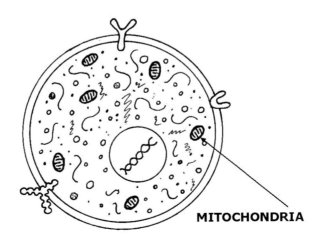

MITOCHONDRIA

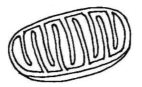

MITOCHONDRIA

The mitochondrial apparatus is used by cholesterol to convert cholesterol to the steroid hormone pregnenolone. Pregnenolone then leaves the mitochondria to go back into the main cell compartment (cytoplasm) to be converted into other steroid hormones.

Medical research has repeatedly demonstrated that the key to systemic health is crucially linked to the mitochondia, which, are also often referred to the powerhouse of the cell. The presence of fewer mitochondria, and/or poor mitochondial health can be directly linked to compromised health.[17,18]

The energy made in the body to carry out any function including breathing, moving, thinking, as well as millions of other functions, is dependent upon the mitochondria for energy in the form of the adenosine triphosphate molecule (ATP). This is why the health of mitochondria is so critical.

Mitochondria are very sensitive to oxidative damage from the general metabolic process as well as environmental damage; for example, cigarette smoke.[19]

The mitochondria also have their own DNA, known as mitochondrial DNA, which is responsible for the production of many important proteins. Recent studies have shown that the mitochondria have steroid hormones receptors, indicating that steroid hormones have a role in mitochondrial action including protein synthesis from the mitochondria's own DNA (mitochondrial DNA).[299]

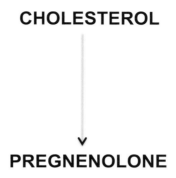

CHOLESTEROL

PREGNENOLONE

This reaction takes place in the mitochondria of the cell.

With aging, cells accumulate metabolic and environmental damage, steroid hormone production slows down and mitochondrial function declines, eventually compromising cell function and health.

How Steroid Hormones Work

Steroid hormones work in complex ways and they work differently from other types of hormones. Where other hormones instruct the cells through cell wall receptors, steroid hormones work in multiple ways.[20,21,22,23,24,25,26,27] For example:

- Steroid hormones can also interact with the cells through the cell wall receptors.

- They can diffuse straight into the cells and interact with receptors in the main part of the cell (cytoplasm).

- They can diffuse into the nucleus of the cell and interact directly with DNA to produce proteins etc.

It is important to recognize that indiscriminate use of steroid hormones can have extensive undesirable consequences.

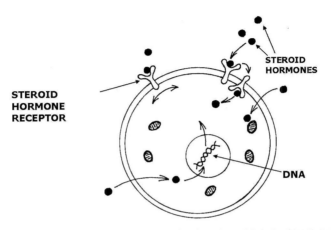

STEROID HORMONE ACTION ON THE CELL

Steroid Hormones in the Brain

The ovaries, testes, and adrenal glands have been known to be the source of steroid hormone synthesis; however, recently it has been found that the brain also synthesizes steroid hormones for its use.[28,29] These hormones are called neurosteroids, and are also produced from cholesterol.[30]

The main neurosteroids are pregnenolone, progesterone, allopregnenolone and dehydroepiandrosterone (DHEA).[31] Very little is known about neurosteroid hormone production or replacement.

Chapter 8

Ovaries

Women are born with two ovaries, which are located in the pelvic region.

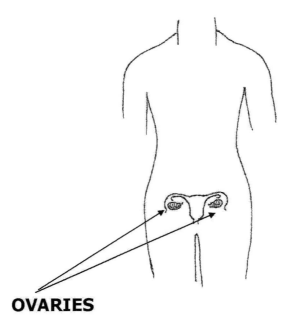

OVARIES

Ovaries are also referred to as gonads (as are testes), and the hormones they produce— estrogen and progesterone—are referred to as gonadal hormones.

Ovaries are responsible for the storage, maturation, and release of eggs. Ovarian hormones are also necessary for the health and normal functioning of the female reproductive system,[32] as well as the development of sexual characteristics and optimal health.

It is estimated that, before birth (at about fifth month of gestation), there are about 7 million potential eggs in the ovary. This number is reduced to about 300,000 at reproductive maturity (near menarche), and less than 1,000 at menopause. A woman typically ovulates about 450 times during her reproductive life.[33]

The first major changes seen in girls are the changes at adrenarche, which is a stage of maturation of the cortex of the adrenal glands. (See Chapter 22, Adrenal Glands.) This usually occurs at an average of age nine. Menarche, the onset of the first menstrual cycle, typically occurs a few years after adrenarche.

How and when a woman sexually develops is determined genetically and is also influenced by the environment.

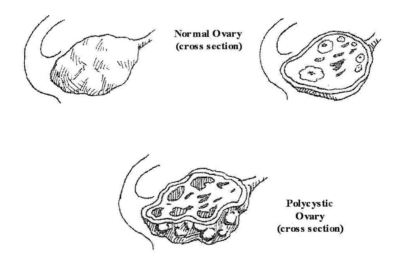

Normal Ovary
(cross section)

Polycystic
Ovary
(cross section)

Brain and Ovary Connection

The brain closely responds to the ovarian hormones throughout a woman's reproductive life. FSH and LH are hormones produced in the brain that stimulate the ovaries to produce estradiol and progesterone.

The normal menstrual cycle relies on this communication. However, what triggers and regulates the menstrual cycle, including input from the adrenal glands and other chemicals, remains to be better understood.

When ovarian function declines due to age, tubal ligation, or surgery, the brain hormones FSH and LH remain elevated. If the ovarian hormones are replaced, these same brain hormones respond by reducing appropriately.

It is on the basis of this communication loop that we predict menopause, ovarian failure, and other aging symptoms.

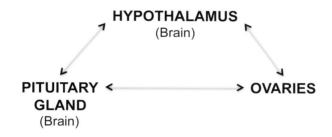

The brain produces hormones that stimulate the ovaries to produce ovarian hormones. These, in turn, regulate many of the brain hormones and chemicals.

Studies have linked premenopausal cardiovascular health to the hormones produced in the brain and ovaries,[34] demonstrating the complex interaction of steroid hormones and other chemical signals to vital health functions.

Production of Hormones from the Ovaries

Maturing ovarian follicles (structures containing an egg) are the main source of hormone production in the ovaries. Other than this, there are several other types of cells within the ovary that produce steroid hormones. This is all conducted in a highly regulated way with specific well-coordinated signals.

After menopause, if the ovaries are still present (i.e., have not been surgically removed), other ovarian cells take over whatever little ovarian hormone production is required.

The ovarian hormones, like all steroid hormones, are derived from cholesterol. The cholesterol used for hormone synthesis comes from at least three different sources:

- The most common is from LDL in the blood. LDL is cholesterol bound to a low-density protein. FSH and LH from the brain cause an increase in the production of LDL receptors (cell gates) so that cholesterol can enter the hormone producing cells.
- Ovaries have the capacity to produce cholesterol from scratch.
- After making and storing cholesterol as lipid droplets, the ovaries can retrieve it as needed.

Other Sources of Sex Hormones in Women

During the reproductive years, the ovaries produce about two-thirds of the total testosterone. The rest is mainly produced in the adrenal glands after androstenedione and DHEA convert to testosterone and estrogens.[35] Testosterone produced in the ovaries converts to estrogen. We are not clear how much, if any, of the testosterone from the ovaries is released into the blood as testosterone before converting to estrogen.

Fat cells and skin cells also make some of the circulating sex hormones. Fat cells have enzymes that convert testosterone to estrogen. Skin cells can use DHEA and androstenedione to make testosterone.[35]

Dihydrotestosterone (DHT) is the most potent androgen. It is thought that in women more than 60 percent of DHT is produced in the skin from the conversion of androstenedione.[35] Androstenedione in women comes mainly from the adrenal glands.

Chapter 9

Menstrual Cycle

The female menstrual cycle is regulated by a complex interaction involving at least the brain (hypothalamus and pituitary), adrenal glands, and the ovaries.

It is the events surrounding the maturation and release of an egg that lead to the cycling hormone production and the menstrual cycle.

We don't fully understand the exact hormones and chemical signals that are involved in fine-tuning the menstrual cycle; however, there is a contribution from progesterone, estrogens, cortisol, as well as corticotropin-releasing hormone (CRH), oxytocin, and others.

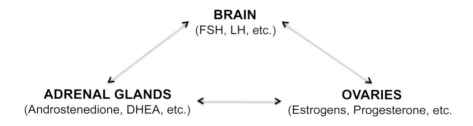

The hypothalamus in the brain releases gonadotropin-releasing hormone (GnRH). GnRH is released in a daily rhythmic pattern, stimulating the pituitary gland (in the brain) to release the hormones FSH and LH.

FSH and LH stimulate the ovaries to release an egg (ovulation). There is a monthly cyclic pattern of release of FSH and LH from the brain. High estrogen inhibits FSH release. Low estrogen stimulates FSH release. Therefore, FSH levels are used as a strong predictor of ovarian function. High baseline FSH reflects ovarian decline.[36]

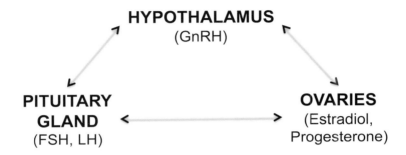

FSH causes an increased production of the enzyme aromatase (CYP19), which converts androstenedione to estrone and testosterone to estradiol.

As mentioned, testosterone is produced in the ovaries, as well as from DHEA and androstenedione from the adrenal glands.

At menopause, there is a high FSH level, as well as more androstenedione from adrenals, leading to higher levels of estrone than were present in youth, which is considered more carcinogenic.

LH at base levels stimulates production of enzymes needed for steroid hormone synthesis. It also stimulates the production of low-density lipoprotein (LDL) and high-density lipoprotein (HDL — "good" cholesterol) receptors; thus preparing the ovaries and adrenal glands for the next cycle of events.

The interplay of LH and FSH to the ovaries for ovulation (release of an egg) is a complex, elegantly orchestrated chain of events.

The role of the adrenal glands, although important, is less clearly understood.

The menstrual cycle is arbitrarily divided into two parts:

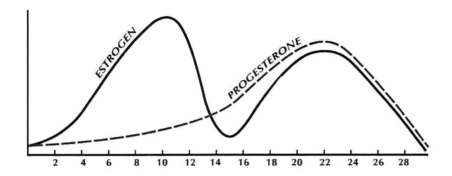

MENSTRUAL CYCLE

The natural cycle of a healthy premenopausal woman is about twenty-eight to thirty-one days, which is similar to the duration of the lunar (moon) cycle. Day one is the first day of bleeding. The first two weeks are known as the follicular phase. During this period, the hormones FSH and LH steadily rise.

Of the many potential follicles capable of maturing and releasing an egg, only one normally becomes the main follicle, which actually releases an egg. The main egg continues to mature, while the others diminish. The second two weeks are known as the luteal phase.

The ovarian cycle and the uterus have always been linked to reproduction. The uterus function, as far as we know, is limited to reproduction, but the ovarian cycle is consistent with the state of fertility and optimum health. Women who do not cycle regularly have health problems, and those who stop cycling—as in menopause—start to age rapidly. The female body is designed to function optimally when the ovarian hormones are produced in the unique rhythm designed by nature.

The Follicular Phase (First Half) of the Menstrual Cycle

The first half of the cycle is called the follicular phase because the egg containing follicle is getting ready to release its egg. The length of this phase varies, and is what determines the length of the overall cycle.

- There is a rapid rise in estradiol production during the first nine to twelve days.

- Estrogen is particularly dose dependant. At each level it initiates a different set of events.

- At an internally determined set point, the brain signals the ovaries to stop producing estrogen, and initiates ovulation (release of an egg).

- It is critical for the brain hormone LH to coordinate its surge with the increasing estrogen for the maturation of the egg as well as numerous other regenerative functions of the body.

- Estrogen levels and rhythm are directly related to a complex network of events in the rest of the body as well as the ovaries.

Luteal Phase (Second Half) of the Menstrual Cycle

The second half of the cycle is led by different set of events that critically determines the health of the individual. The majority of progesterone produced in a fertile woman comes from the structure that released an egg—the *corpus luteum*.

Corpus Luteum

This is the structure that remains after the follicle releases an egg.

A few days after ovulation, the corpus luteum starts to make estrogen and progesterone. The corpus luteum is filled with cholesterol from which it will make these steroid hormones. The life of the corpus luteum is around fourteen days.

For about two weeks, the corpus luteum produces estradiol and progesterone in a rhythm.

The estradiol and progesterone produced from the corpus luteum are usually in proportion to each other as they are made in the same substructure.

The follicle and other parts of the ovary make estradiol in the follicular phase (first half). If the estrogen made in the first half of the cycle is not balanced by the progesterone made in the second half of the cycle, there is a potential for many diseases including premenstrual syndrome (PMS), breast fibroids and cancer, uterine fibroids, and endometrial cancer among others.

The first day of bleeding is considered day one, and has always been thought to occur due to the decline in progesterone production. This view was supported with use of progesterone in birth control pills to induce a period. However, after realizing that women who do not ovulate and therefore do not have a corpus luteum, can still have a regular period (bleeding), it is clear that there are other factors that contribute to regular uterine bleeding/shedding. The mechanisms involved are highly complex and not as well understood as once thought.

Just prior to ovulation, progesterone levels also increase.[37,38] The origin of this progesterone is not clearly understood, but is thought to be linked to the pre-ovulation LH surge, which causes a small amount of progesterone production from the ovaries and adrenal glands. However, it is quite clear that post-ovulatory progesterone is from the corpus luteum.

Different women feel symptomatic at different points in the menstrual cycle. Knowing on what days symptoms occur helps to understand where the problem lies, which helps when considering treatment.

Chapter 10

Estrogen

Estrogen is a steroid hormone, and, like all steroid hormones, it is derived from cholesterol. Ovarian production of estrogens is illustrated in the following graphic.

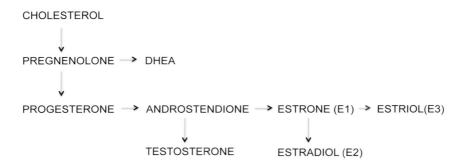

Estrogen is the major sex hormone in females. The major source of estrogen in women is the ovaries. Some amount of estrogen is also produced from the conversion of adrenal androgens.

In males, estrogen also has critical functions and is mostly converted from testosterone. However, the ratio of estrogen to testosterone is much smaller in men than in women.

Types of Estrogen

There are several different types of estrogen; each has a very specific structure and function. The main circulating estrogens in human females are estrone, estradiol and estriol.

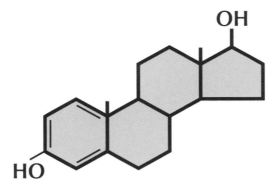

ESTRADIOL *(17B-estradiol)*

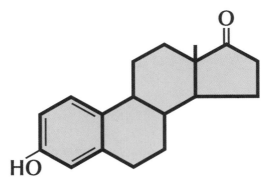

ESTRONE (E$_1$)

ESTRIOL (E$_3$)

Estradiol (E2)

The major estrogen produced by the human ovary is 17-β-estradiol, also referred to as estradiol. Estradiol is the predominant type of estrogen found in premenopausal women.[39] More than 95 percent of estradiol in circulation is produced from the ovaries.[40]

Estrone (E1)

Estrone is also produced in the human ovary, but in very small amounts. Estrone is the predominant form of circulating estrogen after menopause.[39] Of the estrone in the body, only about half comes from the ovaries, where some of it is converted reversibly from estradiol; the rest is converted from androgens (testosterone, androstenedione, DHEA) in tissues such as hair, skin, fat and liver.[40] Estrone is not thought of as favorable because several studies show it to be carcinogenic and inflammatory, especially after it is broken down.

Estriol (E3)

Estriol in non-pregnant women is produced only as an irreversible byproduct (metabolite) of estradiol and estrone. Estriol is thought to be especially useful in the genital and urinary tract tissue where there are estriol receptors. For this reason, it is favored by many physicians for restoring the health of vaginal tissue and for lubrication. But importantly, estriol is a byproduct of estradiol, so if estriol is thought to be deficient, estradiol is most likely also deficient, an important consideration when replacing estrogen.

In pregnancy, especially toward the third trimester, there is a very large amount of estriol in the maternal circulation. This is shown to come from the adrenal glands of the fetus. We do not fully understand why there is so much at that time, but it is likely that it has some use in preparing the birth canal for delivery. Estriol is also the estrogen that the placenta secretes during pregnancy.[39]

Significance of Exact Molecular Structure

The three major estrogens made in the body (estradiol, estrone, and estriol) play some roles that seem to be interchangeable but other roles that are highly specific and not interchangeable.

Steroid hormones are extremely potent chemicals. A one-atom difference in the molecular structure of a hormone makes a critical difference in its function. Also, the body is equipped with enzymes that break down hormones appropriately after they have been used. Hormone-like synthetic chemicals are not recognized or broken down the same way; therefore, they have a longer life, which makes them more potent.

The molecular difference between estradiol and testosterone is just one hydrogen atom. Males convert testosterone to estradiol so it can perform crucial functions in the brain, bones, and other systems. The differences between the synthetic estrogens available for contraception and menopausal symptoms have more molecular differences than just the one atom difference between estradiol and testosterone.

Functions of Estrogen

Estrogen, like all hormones, is a cell-signaling molecule. Because it is a steroid hormone, estrogen can enter and interact with the cell in several different ways. To perform its signaling functions, estrogen requires various helper chemicals, the dynamics of which are extremely complex.

We are still learning about the mechanisms by which estrogen interacts with other hormone systems and molecules to carry out its functions of cell signaling.[41] Research has been going on for several years on the different types of estrogen receptors on different cell types and the implications of these variations.[42,43,44,45,289,298]

Estrogen is unique in how it is produced in a healthy, fertile woman. No hormone is produced in such an elegant distinct pattern as is estrogen. It underlies the function of almost every aspect of female health.

Estrogen creates receptors for other hormones; for example, progesterone, thyroid hormone, and growth hormone. This is one of the important reasons not to add a hormone to the body when there are no receptors for it.

Decline in ovarian function and diminishing estrogen is a gradual process, and produces different symptoms and loss of function in various systems at different levels of decline.

The medical literature provides exhaustive information on the numerous effects of estrogen.

Bone

- Estrogen is critical in bone remodeling and mineralization.[46,47] Estrogens are known to play an important role in regulating bone remodeling and preventing menopausal bone loss.[43,48,49]

- In both genders, estrogen is responsible for the length of long bones.

- Estrogen stimulates calcium resorption from the kidneys and absorption from the small intestines.[50,51]

Brain and Central Nervous System

- Estrogen's activity in the brain is critical to mental functioning. The evidence in the scientific literature regarding the beneficial effects of estrogen on the brain and nervous system is constantly increasing.[52,53,54,55,56,57,58,290] The areas of the brain that specifically respond to estrogen (i.e., have receptors for estrogen) are continuously being discovered.[58]

- The aging brain suffers from changes that can be reversed, slowed down, or halted with the correct replacement of estrogen.

- Males also have estrogen receptors in the brain, and it is thought that testosterone converts to estrogen to respond to these areas.

- Estrogen is involved in higher cognitive functions, susceptibility to seizures, fine motor skills, and mood.[59]

- Estrogen's affect on memory has been well documented. Scientific articles also relate to the neuroprotection of estrogen in stroke as well as in neurodegenerative diseases such as Parkinson's disease and Alzheimer's disease.[59,60,61,62]

- The interactions of various neurotransmitters, including serotonin, are tightly linked to estrogen levels.

- When the results of the Women's Health Initiative (WHI) Study were released in 2002, many physicians took women off Prempro® (a prescription hormone replacement therapy product) and other hormones and offered antidepressants instead. Any positive effect of the antidepressants was due to the antidepressant's effects on the brain's serotonin activity, which mimics some of the estrogen effects. However, this was not a good long-term choice.

- Depression is highly linked to estrogen balance.[52] It is more medically sound to perform a thorough hormone balance check in women who complain of depression before considering antidepressants.

- Estrogen regulates other brain hormones including LH, FSH, thyroid-stimulating hormone (TSH), growth hormone, and prolactin, as well as numerous neurotransmitters.

- Estrogen levels and balance are linked to sensation of pain.[52] It is common for menstruating women to feel pain in parts of the cycle during which estrogen is low. The mechanism is complex and appears to be linked to estrogen's effect on neurotransmitters and neurotransmitter receptors.

- Several research studies have linked migraine headaches to hormone imbalance.[45,63,64] More research is needed in this area to clarify the imbalance.

The entire explanation of how estrogen affects the brain is exhaustive and complex with still a lot to be learned. It is clear, however, that there is a strong connection between brain function and estrogen balance.

Breasts

- Estrogen is well known to have effects on the development of breasts,[44] and a balance is needed to maintain healthy breast tissue.

- Progesterone down-regulates estrogen receptors. This is important in the ovarian cycle. If progesterone is not produced adequately, estrogen receptors are not down-regulated, and breast tissue can grow out of balance leading to problems such as fibrous tissue, and benign and malignant tumors. (See Chapter 17, Breast and Ovarian Cancer)

Cardiovascular System

The positive effects of estrogen on the cardiovascular system cannot be escaped. It was the basis for landmark studies such as the WHI study and the Heart and Estrogen/Progestin Replacement Study (HERS). Those studies were badly designed (as we will discuss later), and discredited thousands of studies done before them. They also created doubt in the studies done after them.

- The cardiovascular system is dependent on the correct levels of estrogen.[65] This observation interested scientists decades ago, when they realized that, after menopause, women's incidence of heart disease was similar to that in men, while, during their years of balanced estrogen, they appeared relatively protected.

- Men have more cardiovascular protection when treated with testosterone. It is not clear how much of this is due to the direct effects of testosterone versus the effects of estradiol after testosterone converts to it.

- Estrogen has an important role in the integrity of blood vessels of all sizes, including the body's ability to create new blood vessels.[51,66]

- Blood pressure is reduced by the correct balance of estrogen. Estrogen promotes vasodilation (relaxation) of blood vessels by increasing the production of nitric oxide.[51] Estrogen also reduces blood pressure by its effects on other proteins.[67,68] Blood pressure has been demonstrated to decrease with transdermal estrogen replacement.[68]

- There are estrogen receptors on the walls of blood vessels. In multiple ways, these receptors facilitate healthy functioning and hence protection from cardiovascular disease.[45,65,69,70,71,72,73,291] Estrogen is well known to have anti-atherogenic effects (prevents plaque from sticking to arteries) in men and women.[175] High-frequency ultrasound measurements have demonstrated the cardioprotective effects of estrogen on blood vessel walls.[74]

- The blood vessel walls also need estrogenic effects to prevent calcification from the deregulation of bone mineralization, which occurs in the absence of adequate estrogen.[75]

- Estrogen has been demonstrated to have blood pressure lowering effects by improving the tone and reducing the stress in arteries.[45] The mechanisms are numerous and complex. Of note, this advantage is not seen with synthetic estrogen.

- Studies have also demonstrated that the heart muscle cells also have estrogen receptors. A study in Germany suggested that this could contribute to the gender-based differences in cardiac function.[77]

- The role of estrogen was investigated in survival after a coronary artery bypass surgery in postmenopausal women. Women who had been on hormone replacement therapy were shown to have a significantly greater in-hospital survival.[78]

- Studies have also shown that women who had been on estrogen replacement therapy had a better hospital survival after a myocardial infarction than those who never had estrogen replacement.[79]

Clotting of Blood

- The balance of estrogen is crucial for the correct clotting of blood.[52] Both high and low levels of estrogen have been associated with increased blood clots, leading to thromboembolism (a blood clot dislodging and causing a blockage in some other artery).[52]

- Several studies have shown that replacement of estrogen in postmenopausal women reduces the incidence of stroke.[79,80]

- Women on birth control pills are at risk for blood clots, as mentioned on the package inserts.

- Synthetic estrogens in birth control pills are much more potent than bioidentical estrogens because the body is not equipped to break down foreign molecules as it does its own.

- Estrogen by mouth enters the liver before it gets into general circulation. A daily dose of by-mouth estrogen triggers the liver to make proteins such as blood clotting proteins. A product applied topically enters the general circulation before it enters the liver. (Synthetic progesterone is also thought to have an adverse affect on blood clots as demonstrated in the WHI study)

- It is common to see postmenopausal women take longer to stop bleeding after a needle stick and to bruise more.

Energy and Mitochondria

- Estrogen receptors have been demonstrated to exist on the mitochondria, suggesting that estrogen has critical effects on mitochondrial functioning.[16,20,81,82,83,84,85]

- Women and men both report experiencing more energy after hormone replacement.

Fat

Estrogen decreases adipose (fat) tissue by stimulating the enzymes that break down fat. Loss of estrogen results in fat accumulation in adipose tissue (fat cells), especially in the abdomen.[51]

Growth

Estrogens are key regulators of growth, differentiation, and correct functioning of many tissues, including structures of the male and female reproductive tract, skeletal system, breast tissue, nerve tissue, cardiovascular system, digestive system, and immune systems.[59]

Growth Hormone

- Estrogen is well recognized to be involved in the secretion of growth hormone from the brain (See Chapter 25 Growth Hormone).[86,87]

- Growth hormone is released from the brain in a pulsatile manner. After menopause, growth hormone secretion declines. This is thought to be due in part to the decline in estrogen.

Hair

- Women experience healthier hair growth on the scalp when the estrogen cycle is in balance. The hair generally becomes thicker, and grows longer with an improved texture.

- Interesting work has been done to show improvement of hair growth with local application of estrogen;[89] however, further studies are needed to determine the long-term consequences for such a use.

Immune System

Estrogen—specifically estradiol—is involved in balancing the immune system.[52,90]

- In the immune system, estrogen's main effect is as an immune suppressor,[52] which means that it prevents the body from attacking itself.

- Many age-related autoimmune diseases that have a genetic component manifest after perimenopause and menopause when estrogen levels are low; for example, systemic lupus erythematosus.[91,92]

- It is thought that, in a low-estrogen environment, the body is in attack mode, and any predisposition to disease can be brought out; however, more studies are needed to substantiate this.

- Interestingly, during the progression of pregnancy, when estrogen levels are extraordinarily high, it is beneficial to the fetus that the mother's immune system is not "hostile" toward it.

- After delivery, estrogen levels drop; this helps the mother, who needs a strong immune system to protect against delivery trauma, and to ensure plentiful antibodies in the milk she produces for the newborn.

Lipid Profile and Cholesterol

As we have seen, cholesterol is essential for life; however, it needs to be utilized.

- Estrogen is instrumental in ensuring that the cell wall is correctly constructed so that cholesterol, as well as other necessary molecules, can enter.

- Estrogen facilitates cholesterol entry into the cells by stimulating production of LDL receptors, which are necessary for the entry of cholesterol in the form of LDL.[51,52] This helps to ensure that cholesterol stays within healthy blood levels.

- Numerous studies have demonstrated that estrogen benefits the lipid profile and decreases atherosclerosis.[93]

- The luteal phase of the menstrual cycle, which has high levels of estrogen , has been shown to be associated with a decrease in the risk of coronary artery disease.[94] The exact mechanism is not clear.

- The Lipid Research Clinics Program Follow-up Study followed 2270 women aged forty to sixty-nine for an average of eight and a half years to determine the effects of estrogen on heart disease. The results showed estrogen to be statistically significant in the protection against heart disease.[95]

Liver

Estrogen stimulates the liver to produce a variety of proteins, many of which are needed to carry and transport other hormones.

- Special proteins are needed to facilitate the entry of estrogen into the cells.[52] Without adequate levels of these special proteins, estrogen cannot carry out many of its functions.

- The liver's production of these proteins is tightly regulated by the dose of estrogen. This is one of the reasons that taking oral estrogen can be hazardous, as it stimulates abnormal levels of certain proteins due to an artificially high level of estrogen.

Skin

- The skin contains estrogen receptors which facilitate improvement in many ways;[89,96] for example, estrogen increases the collagen content of the skin, increases thickness, and improves moisture retention.[97]

- Some women apply estrogen directly to the face skin to stimulate fibroblasts (special cells in the skin that make collagen and elastic tissue). Although applying estrogen directly to the face may seem beneficial, it is more advisable to balance estrogen internally so the entire body system can benefit.

- At menopause there is a change in the skin. Depending on how the adrenal glands respond after ovarian decline the skin can react in various ways. For example, if there is a strong adrenal response there can be increased oil production, acne or beard area hair growth. If the adrenal response is low, the skin becomes dry and wrinkly.

- Studies have shown urticaria (itchy skin) to be related to changes in the hormonal cycle.[98]

Sleep

Menopausal women commonly complain of sleep disorders independent of hot flashes.

- Sleep-disordered breathing is more common after menopause.[99]

- Estrogen is closely linked to the functions of the neurotransmitter serotonin. Serotonin converts to melatonin in the absence of light.[52] With estrogen depletion, the balance of neurotransmitters and hormones is altered, which could adversely affect restful sleep.

Skeletal Muscle

Estrogen is documented to have a beneficial effect on the skeletal muscles of both men and women.[100]

Thyroid Function

Estrogen has an important role in thyroid hormone function. The mechanism by which estrogen acts at the cellular level in the brain is highly complex. Estrogen increases the sensitivity of the cells in the brain that respond to Thyrotropin-releasing hormone (TRH) causing them to effectively release thyroid-stimulating hormone (TSH), which stimulates the thyroid gland to make and release thyroid hormone.[101]

Urogenital Tract

- The vaginal lining is notably receptive to estrogen. Vaginal dryness is directly proportional to decreased estrogen production. The entire urinary and genital tract has been shown to have estrogen receptors.[44]

- Estriol is not produced by the human ovary. However, estradiol which is the main estrogen produced in the ovaries, irreversibly converts to estriol. The urogenital system (urinary tract structures and genital tract structures) has abundant receptors for estriol.

- It is on this basis that estriol is often given as a vaginal supplement (in suppository form) by many anti-aging physicians. Of note is that firstly, there is no rhythm with estriol suppositories, so long-term consequences are not known. Secondly, if there is vaginal dryness, it is an indication that the body's overall levels of estrogen are low, and other places in the body also need to be addressed.

- Oncologists (cancer specialists) may give estriol to treat vaginal dryness in breast cancer patients. This is with the understanding that estriol should not convert to either estrone or estradiol, both of which have receptors in the breast tissue.

Uterus

- The uterus is the organ most recognized to respond to estrogen. The health and function of the uterus, as well as the events of pregnancy and the menstrual cycle, depend on the levels and pattern of estrogen production.

- Too much estrogen without balanced progesterone causes uterine fibroids and dysfunctional bleeding.

- Estrogen is responsible for uterine wall contractions.

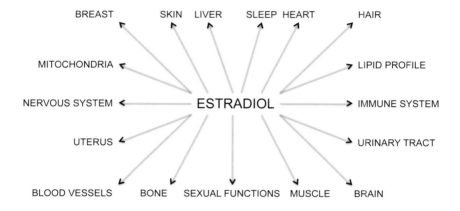

Estrogen-like Molecules

A healthy, fertile woman produces estrogen in a highly regular pattern, dose, and rhythm.

Estrogen is one of the most sophisticated hormones of the human system. Its exact molecular structure and concentration are critical to how it functions in different situations. There is so much we clearly do not understand.

There are many substances—natural and synthetic— which resemble the estrogen molecule and mimic some of its important actions. However, there are fewer similarities than there are differences. When replacing estrogen, it is not medically justifiable to replace it with anything other than what is molecularly identical to what the body makes.

Some of these hazardous synthetic estrogen-like molecules:

- Can be found in birth control pills.

- Can be found in hormones developed for menopausal symptoms. The sources are usually natural; for example, plants and pregnant horses' urine.

- Can be ingested through the food we eat and drink which was treated with hormones to make the food bigger and grow faster.

- Can be found in petrochemicals that leak into drinks and food from containers that they were stored in. These were not designed for replacing estrogen, and are called xenoestrogens.

Metabolism (Breakdown) of Estrogens

Estrogens are carefully metabolized (broken down) by specific enzymes. They are not designed to exist beyond a certain length of time; specific enzymes circulate ready to break down estrogens. The different estrogens that occur naturally in the body (estradiol, estrone, and estriol) are broken (metabolized) down into different byproducts (metabolites). We do not understand how synthetic estrogens are broken. We do know that synthetic estrogens are much more potent than bioidentical hormones because they continue to exist without being eliminated the same way as bioidentical hormones are.

When the body is exposed to estrogen-like molecules, the potential for disruption of balance and health hazards is immeasurable.

Chapter 11

Progesterone

Progesterone is a steroid hormone made from cholesterol.

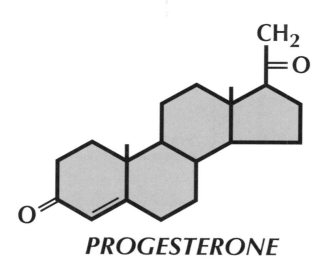

PROGESTERONE

Progesterone is critical for stable health in men and women. Although it is mostly recognized for its role in keeping the tissue of the uterus (endometrium) healthy, progesterone has numerous other roles which are far more important and indispensable. The menopausal body can survive without a uterus, but the rest of the body, including the brain and heart, are more significant for life and depend on progesterone for health.

The ratio and production of progesterone in relation to estrogen and testosterone may vary in men and women, but its role in overall health is essential in both.

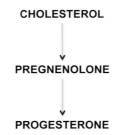

CHOLESTEROL

PREGNENOLONE

PROGESTERONE

Progesterone has many direct effects of its own in hormone balance; it is also converted into other important hormones.

Like all steroid hormones, progesterone can affect cell function in many ways. For example, it can initiate a signal through the cell wall receptors, as well go directly into the cell, or go straight to the DNA to initiate protein synthesis.[102]

Healthy, fertile women mainly release progesterone from the ovaries for fourteen days out of a twenty-eight-to-thirty-one-day cycle.

Although men and women both make progesterone in the adrenal glands and brain, the pattern or rhythm is not well understood.

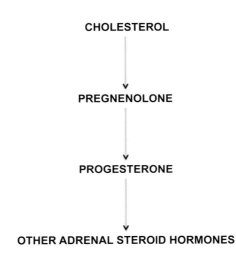

CHOLESTEROL

PREGNENOLONE

PROGESTERONE

OTHER ADRENAL STEROID HORMONES

Simplified diagram of adrenal androgen production

In the pathway of steroid hormone synthesis, progesterone production occurs relatively early. It is likely that progesterone has a baseline level in the blood, which is probably regulated through the adrenal glands, but little data is available to verify the quantity or pattern.

Progesterone in Men

Progesterone is also produced in the testes in the steps towards testosterone production:

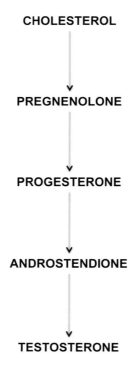

CHOLESTEROL

PREGNENOLONE

PROGESTERONE

ANDROSTENDIONE

TESTOSTERONE

Simplified diagram of steps in males testes androgen production

The pattern of production of progesterone from the male testes is not known; it has not been studied very extensively. There are some studies that are looking at progesterone's role in prostate health.

Progesterone in Women

The production of progesterone in women is much more clearly defined than it is in men. As mentioned above, a healthy, cycling woman produces progesterone for fourteen days out of her monthly cycle.

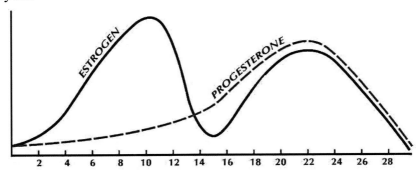

MENSTRUAL CYCLE

The steady rise in estradiol has many functions, one of which is signaling cells to make progesterone receptors.[103]

During the First Half of the Menstrual Cycle

The rising estradiol reaches a critical high on about day twelve. Ovulation is triggered, and estradiol production declines. Again, one of the important functions of the rising estradiol is to create progesterone receptors.

Mid-cycle and Beyond

* LH (luteinizing hormone) from the brain stimulates the ripened ovarian follicle to release an egg (ovulation).

* The corpus luteum (the remnant of the ovarian follicle that

just released an egg) normally produces a balanced amount of estrogen and progesterone for about two weeks.

If this does not take place correctly hormone imbalance occurs, which can lead to many different symptoms, including infertility. If conception occurs, the placenta produces progesterone to sustain the pregnancy.[53] One of the common reasons to miscarry is due to inadequate progesterone produced by the placenta.

Functions of Progesterone

Progesterone balances the effects of estrogen, as well as having countless critical functions of its own. It is also a precursor to almost all steroid hormones. The medical literature is full of information describing the different functions of progesterone in the human body other than its commonly recognized role in the uterus. One of the most interesting roles of progesterone recognized recently is its importance in balancing brain function.[104]

Brain

- Progesterone has calming effects on the brain, and balances the effects of estrogen. The absence of progesterone after estrogen stimulation can promote agitation, anxiety, and restlessness—typically seen with PMS.

- During the anovulatory years, when there is inadequate progesterone due to menstruation without the release of an egg, women feel the most PMS symptoms.

- Progesterone withdrawal in the menstrual cycle has been linked to enhanced seizure susceptibility. Studies are ongoing to determine the role of progesterone-like steroids (neurosteroids) for seizure control.[106,107]

- Progesterone acts on the brain in thermoregulation (body temperature control) by elevating body temperature. This is why body temperature can be used to determine if ovulation occurred.[52]

- Progesterone acts on the brain's response to carbon dioxide levels for respiration.[51]

- Progesterone has been shown to be neuroprotective after brain trauma in numerous studies. It is being further investigated for treatment after stroke and brain injury[108] as well as spinal cord injury.[109,110] Although progesterone has been demonstrated to be neuroprotective,[111] the synthetic progesterone Provera® (medroxyprogesterone acetate, or MPA) does not offer neuroprotection, but instead, is reported to antagonize the positive effects of estrogen,[63,287] making the nervous system vulnerable to degenerative insults.[112]

Breasts

- Progesterone is necessary for maintaining healthy breast tissue and complementing the tissue building effects of estrogen. Although women can have fibrous nodules in their breasts at any time in their life, they are most commonly seen in the early menstrual years, when it is most common to have anovulatory cycles (menstruation without release of an egg, and therefore absence of the progesterone phase). It is necessary to replace progesterone with bioidentical progesterone only, and in a natural cyclic dose. Synthetic progesterone in a continuous dose has detrimental effects on breast tissue.[113]

- Women who have high estrogen with low progesterone for extended cycles are at a greater risk for breast cancer.

- During the perimenopause years when women do not ovulate well, there is a greater risk for breast cancer and possibly other cancers from inadequate amounts of progesterone to balance the estrogen.

- Estrogen alone is not the risk factor for breast cancer. It is estrogen without progesterone balance that causes unregulated tissue growth with greater chances of mutations leading to cancer. (See Chapter 17, Breast And Ovarian Cancer)

Cardiovascular

Progesterone is cardioprotective. It is important to know that progesterone and not any of its synthetic derivatives including medroxyprogesterone acetate, (MPA, also sold under the trade name Provera®) has beneficial effects on the walls of blood vessels.[74,295]

Kidneys

Progesterone acts on the kidneys to help eliminate salt and water.[51] Women often feel bloated when their progesterone is not correctly balanced with estrogen.

Skin

Along with estrogen, progesterone is important for the integrity of the skin because it increases collagen synthesis and stops the enzymes that break down collagen.[51]

Uterus and Ovaries

Balancing the uterus from estrogen exposure is the most medically recognized function of progesterone.[113] Recognizing this function while disregarding how critical it is elsewhere, resulted in landmark studies such as the Women's Health Initiative Study where thousands of women were placed on estrogen without progesterone, just because they did not have a uterus.

- Without adequate progesterone, pregnancy cannot advance because the uterus cannot be prepared for the implantation of an embryo.

- Many women have trouble maintaining a pregnancy

because of inadequate progesterone produced from the corpus luteum or the uterus.[53]Progesterone therapy can help women retain the fetus and protect the pregnancy.

- Progesterone is required for the proper cycling of the uterus lining. Without progesterone, the uterus growth is unregulated, which results in a myriad of uterine dysfunctions not limited to endometriosis and uterine fibroids. There is a greater risk of endometrial cancer without adequate progesterone.[116]

- Countless hysterectomies have been performed because of uterine dysfunctions resulting from abnormal estrogen and progesterone balance.

- Traditional medical belief is that progesterone withdrawal signals the initiation of a period; however, the evidence is conflicting. Women who do not ovulate, for example, in the first and last few years of the menstrual years, do not produce the cyclic luteal phase progesterone, but still bleed regularly. Also, many women with polycystic ovaries have very regular periods regardless of the absence of correct progesterone cycling.

- Other hormones, including those from the adrenal glands and the brain, have a critical role in regulating the menstrual cycle, but their exact role is not understood well at this time.

- Progesterone has an important role in regulating the various cells of the ovaries.[116,117,118] The implication of this is significant when considering ovarian dysfunction and infertility.

Synthetic Progesterone

Provera® is the trade name for medroxyprogesterone acetate (MPA), the most common form of synthetic progesterone used for menopausal women.

MPA is also the synthetic version of progesterone used in the Women's Health Initiative (WHI) Study and the Heart and Estrogen/ Progesterone Replacement Study (HERS). The results of these studies created the controversy over hormone replacement therapy. (See Chapter 16)

It is important to understand that MPA is not the same as the progesterone made in the human body. In many critical areas of the body, including the cardiovascular system, MPA has been shown to have negative effects.[112,119]

Where bioidentical progesterone compliments and balances the effects of estradiol, the consequences of MPA are significantly unfavorable and counteract the beneficial effects of the body's natural estrogen (estradiol) .[120,121,122,123,124]

Several different types of cell receptors exist, which interact with progesterone and progesterone-like molecules in complex mechanisms.[125] Steroids communicate with cells in elaborate mechanisms, which we are just beginning to understand. Also, steroid effects are concentration dependant, which adds to their complex dynamics. It is medically unsound to supplement the body with a synthetic version of any steroid hormone, especially one so critical to health, and especially when bioidentical versions are available.

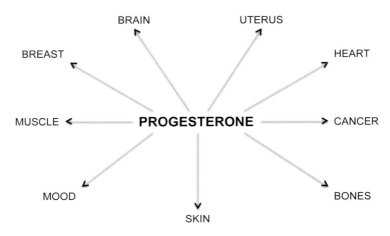

Chapter 12

Menopause and Perimenopause

Perimenopause

Perimenopause is a state of hormone imbalance caused by the ovarian function beginning to decline. As a woman's ovaries age, there is a decline in the amount of estrogen produced throughout the monthly cycles. The mid-cycle estradiol peak is not as high, and if ovulation does occur, adequate progesterone and estrogen are not produced.

Every woman experiences perimenopause differently. The process typically starts about ten years before menopause. If a woman has used birth control pills or has had other ovarian disturbances, perimenopause starts earlier than genetically predicted.

Perimenopausal women experience many of the following symptoms:

- Mood and anxiety disorders

- Often more PMS symptoms

- Irregular and often painful menstrual cycles

- Changes in the pattern and quality of the menstrual cycle; for example, shorter or longer interval, and heavier bleeding first few days of the cycle, with a quick tapering off

- Painful breasts often with nodules

- Thinning skin, hair, and nails

- Oily skin and pimples around the chin area

- More difficulty in losing weight, with a change in body

build and constitution

- Changes in memory

- Changes in thyroid function (estrogen has direct and indirect effects on thyroid function)

- Changes in sexual function and interest

Many other changes take place in the body without producing symptoms; for example:

- Osteoporosis usually begins

- Lipid profile begins to change as less cholesterol enters cells

- Hormone levels in other systems change: thyroid, insulin, growth hormone, and others

- Central nervous system changes

- Muscle mass start to decline

- Immune system is affected

Every organ system is affected with hormone decline. Hormones are cell signals; if they do not function adequately, cells cannot function optimally, and the overall health declines.

Menopause

Clinical Diagnosis

A woman is said to have reached menopause when she has had no menstrual period for one year. The average age of menopause is fifty-one. There is a strong genetic component to the age at which menopause occurs, but is also influenced by environmental components such as those that affect the onset of perimenopause; for example, birth control pills, medications, cigarette smoking, and other factors.

- Menopause is a gradual process caused by the aging of the ovaries.

- It is typical for a woman to experience menstrual irregularity months to years before menopause is officially diagnosed.

- The time between healthy ovarian cycling and menopause is called perimenopause.

- All the symptoms of perimenopause can occur at menopause but are usually more severe.

- Although the symptoms of menopause vary among women, most women have common symptoms such as hot flashes and night sweats.

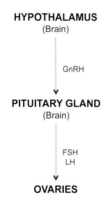

At menopause the ovary-to-brain communication changes:

- The ovarian hormones (estradiol and progesterone) are very low with negligible cycling.

- Because progesterone and estradiol levels are low, LH and FSH are not suppressed and remain constantly elevated.

- When menopause is suspected, physicians typically measure FSH and LH. If the levels are above a certain criteria, the diagnosis of menopause is confirmed.

Physical Changes

Women gradually start to lose their youthful femininity near menopause. The female cycle of estrogen and progesterone is gone, and the hormonal makeup of youth is replaced by a different ratio of hormones.

If the adrenal glands are healthy, they "compensate" the low ovarian function and operate on a different set of terms. DHEA made from the adrenal glands converts to testosterone after entering the general circulation. The balance of estradiol, progesterone, and testosterone changes and women become less feminine.

Women typically experience:

- Changes in hair pattern and thickness on the scalp

- Changes in the voice, which usually becomes slightly deeper

- Appearance of chin and neck hair

- Oily skin and/or acne

- Change in figure and body fat distribution

- Slight coarsening of facial features, especially in the nose and brow area

The medical literature is not consistent on where the testosterone in menopausal women comes from—ovaries or adrenal glands (from DHEA). However, it is clinically seen that women who have had their ovaries removed prior to natural menopause respond in a similar way to those who enter menopause naturally due to aging ovaries. This indicates a strong adrenal role.

Chapter 13

Polycystic Ovary Syndrome

Older medical texts refer to polycystic ovary syndrome as the Stein Leventhal syndrome because it was originally described by Stein and Leventhal in the 1930s. The symptoms of polycystic ovary syndrome are variable and are mainly due to the excess production of androgens (mainly testosterone), as well as dysfunctional ovaries devoid of regular cycling estradiol and progesterone. Cases of polycystic ovary syndrome have dramatically increased over the last fifteen years; however, traditional medicine has still not understood how to treat this disease adequately.

Part of the problem is that so much is not understood about the polycystic ovary syndrome. For example, we are not certain about the origin of the disease—does it start from ovary or adrenal dysfunction? We also do not know if other systems such as the brain or thyroid have any role to play.

It is usual for the adrenal glands to increase DHEA production when the ovaries are not correctly producing estradiol and progesterone in the natural cycling rhythm. Again, the communication network is so complex that we have not determined how the brain, adrenal glands, and ovaries regulate each other.

Symptoms

Some women have polycystic ovaries for years without any obvious symptoms, and are often diagnosed incidentally; for example, during an infertility workup. Others have all the classic symptoms, which are supported by laboratory blood analysis. The most common symptoms are:

- Hirsutism (facial hair especially in chin, cheeks, and neck area)

- Weight gain

- Irregular menstrual cycle, which can worsen to a temporary or permanent termination of the menstrual cycle

- Difficulty conceiving and infertility

- Acne

Along with these symptoms, polycystic ovary syndrome has been linked to coronary heart disease, insulin resistance, diabetes, thyroid dysfunction, adrenal dysfunction, and the metabolic syndrome (a combination of disorders, including insulin resistance, abnormal lipid profile, high blood pressure, excess fat and increased chances for cardiovascular disease).[126,127,128,129]

Polycystic ovary syndrome also leads to a higher risk of breast cancer due the conversion of the testosterone to the less desirable estrogen (estrone) without adequate protection from progesterone.

Diagnosis

Most women in the initial stages of polycystic ovary syndrome do not have any symptoms. As the disease progresses, the presentation of the disease, symptoms, laboratory blood analysis, and ultrasound results vary, so there is no single, reliable diagnostic method.

Traditionally, the method of diagnosis has been to identify two of the following three conditions:

- Amenorrhea (absent menstrual cycle)

- Excess androgen secretion (as evidenced by excess facial hair and acne)

- Polycystic ovaries on ultrasound

Ultrasound measurements can be very useful as a diagnostic, as can the standard measurements of the brain hormones LH and FSH, which, if they exist in an abnormal ratio, can confirm a diagnosis.

However, the problems with standard diagnosing techniques are:

- The classic lab tests could be predictably abnormal to completely normal.

- The ultrasound can show a variety of disease stages, as well as missing fibrous ovaries.

Possible Underlying Causes

There are no studies to confirm what has triggered the tremendous increase in the cases of polycystic ovary syndrome. We are also seeing that girls are getting their period years before their mothers and grandmothers did.

The constant exposure to unwanted hormones and other chemicals that women have been exposed to from birth is thought to have interfered with their normal hormonal balance. For example:

- Hormones are used in the food industry to make larger animals and higher milk production, such as dairy products and meats.

- Contamination occurs from petrochemicals in plastics typically used to store and heat food. Girls who were born after the seventies have had a greater exposure to plastics and petrochemicals than the previous generations due to the conveniences of modern times. As infants, they drank their milk from plastic instead of glass bottles, and the bottles were fitted with newer types of plastic nipples. The milk was also modified to sit longer in the bottle, which then was microwave heated resulting in further insult from petrochemical contamination from the heated plastic.

Prior to Treatment

Before initiating any treatment, it is necessary to get a maximum understanding as to what is happening in the body. For example:

- Determine which hormones, and in which patterns and doses, are being produced by the ovaries.

- If there is a menstrual cycle, conduct a blood test on day ten to see how much estrogen is produced. Although estrogen typically peaks around day twelve, it drops normally very soon after it peaks, so, in case a woman has a short estrogen phase (follicular phase), it is important not to miss the rise completely and get a false low.

- Conduct a second blood test on day twenty-one to determine if there has been ovulation and, if so, how much estrogen and progesterone are produced.

- Conduct a blood test any time between days fourteen and twenty-one of the menstrual cycle to measure free and total testosterone as well as DHEAS to evaluate adrenal function.

Note: If there is no menstrual cycle, then adrenal and ovarian tests can be done any time.

Diet

Nutritional literature recommends that patients with polycystic ovary syndrome follow a type II diabetic diet, which focuses on complex carbohydrates. Anti-inflammatory products such as omega 3 and vitamin E are encouraged, and "bad fats" are discouraged.[126]

Treatment of Polycystic Ovary Syndrome

The ovaries in polycystic ovary syndrome could normalize spontaneously after a few months or continue to worsen. Standard medical treatments for polycystic ovarian syndrome are:

- Spironolactone
- Birth control pills

Treatment with Spironolactone

Spironolactone is a pharmaceutical drug (marketed under several trade names) that is prescribed with the assumption that the cause of polycystic ovary syndrome is excess adrenal production of DHEA, leading to excess circulating testosterone.

Although spironolactone does limit the adrenal production of DHEA and therefore testosterone, it also limits the production of aldosterone, which can lead to low blood pressure, other heart problems, and also disrupt the potassium and electrolyte balance.

In treating polycystic ovary syndrome with spironolactone, the underlying problem is not usually solved, and the side effects can be problematic.

Treatment with Birth Control Pills

Although birth control pills can be an effective method of controlling the symptoms of polycystic ovaries, the underlying problem, again, is usually not solved, and the body is exposed to harmful hormone-mimicking chemicals. (See Chapter 14, Birth Control Pills)

Birth control pills control symptoms of excess testosterone by two possible mechanisms:

- Taking estrogen by mouth triggers the liver to increase production of proteins called sex hormone binding globulin (SHBG). These proteins preferentially bind to free circulating testosterone, reducing the effects of testosterone. The total level of testosterone is not reduced; it is only bound up, therefore "inactive". When the birth control pill is stopped, SHBG production decreases, releasing the testosterone, causing symptoms such as more acne, facial hair, and others.

- When estrogen and progesterone are administered, the brain is not signaled to release the hormones LH and FSH; therefore, the ovaries are not stimulated to produce estradiol and progesterone. The adrenal connection is not fully understood.

Other Possible Options for Treatment

What We Know and Don't Know

We do not fully understand how polycystic ovary syndrome begins. So far, there are no treatments proven to be safe, and the present FDA-approved treatments have harmful side effects. We do know that, if left untreated, polycystic ovaries can lead to other hormonal disturbances and dysfunctions.

We recognize that in polycystic ovaries there is a lack of coordination and balance between the hormones from the brain, adrenal glands, and ovaries.

Historically, it has been observed that many women with polycystic ovaries who become pregnant develop normal ovarian function after delivery. It is speculated that the ovaries were quiet for nine months and not stimulated by the brain hormones (FSH, LH).

A Simpler, Natural Approach

Until we understand the polycystic ovary syndrome better, and acquire more scientific data, we can use the knowledge we have to try a safer approach. If we mimic normal, healthy ovary function, the brain will receive the correct signals and not release excessive LH and FSH, which cause too much ovarian stimulation, and therefore cysts. The cycling ovarian hormones may regulate the adrenal glands so they will not produce excess DHEA, which converts to testosterone, creating the multiple symptoms of polycystic ovaries. By applying topical estrogen and progesterone in the ovarian dose and pattern:

- The rest of the body will get the benefits of the ovarian hormone production.

- The uterus will cycle normally, reducing the risk of endometrial tissue pathology such as fibroids.

- The external hormones will indicate to the brain that the ovaries are producing satisfactory levels of estradiol and progesterone so it can stop releasing high levels of LH and FSH.

- Normalizing the complex brain to ovary communication may adjust the adrenal hormone production to a more natural pattern.

Expected Reactions of Hormone Treatment

Whenever there is a shift in the body's hormone balance, there can be some initial unpredictable reactions by the body, which usually subside if the treatment is continued and the body stays in balance.

For example, women can lose some scalp hair after the high levels of pregnancy hormones are reduced several weeks after delivery. A similar phenomenon can be observed when women shift from unbalanced hormones from dysfunctional ovaries to the normal ovarian rhythm. These, as well as other changes, typically resolve once the body is in balance.

Cautions

It is important to monitor blood levels every few months to ensure correct hormone balance and levels.

Most physicians are not trained to treat polycystic ovaries with anything other than spironolactone or birth control pills; therefore, it is important to only work with physicians who have a thorough understanding of the current scientific medical literature.

Chapter 14

Birth Control Pills

Before a woman considers taking birth control pills, she should be aware of how they work as well as the possible risks and side effects.

What Are They Supposed To Do?

The function of birth control pills is to prevent conception, although, they are also often used to regulate the menstrual cycle and in the treatment of the symptoms of polycystic syndrome.

What Are They?

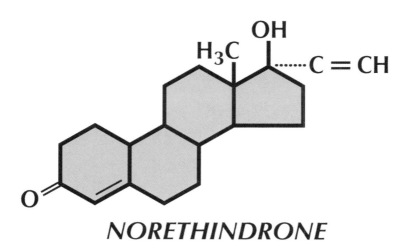

NORETHINDRONE

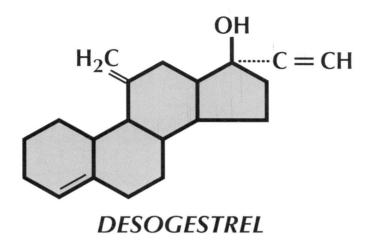

DESOGESTREL

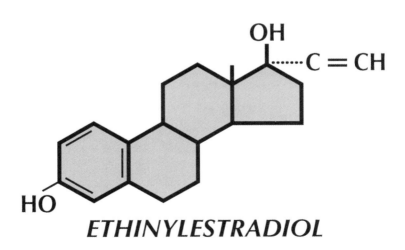

ETHINYLESTRADIOL

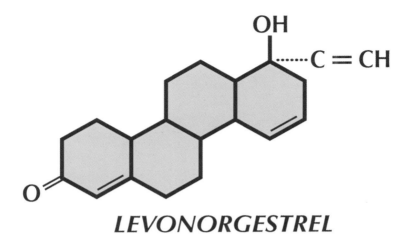

LEVONORGESTREL

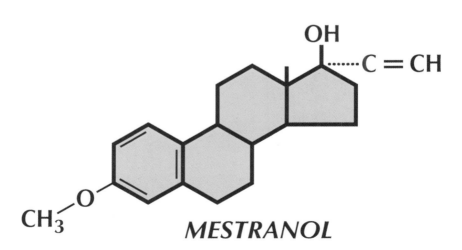

MESTRANOL

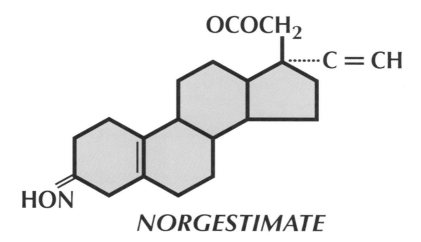

NORGESTIMATE

Birth control pills are typically synthetic versions of estrogen and progesterone. Because these substances are very similar in structure to the body's own estrogen and progesterone, they attach to a lot of the same receptors that the real hormones do and trigger a response.

The following chart illustrates how birth control pills work:

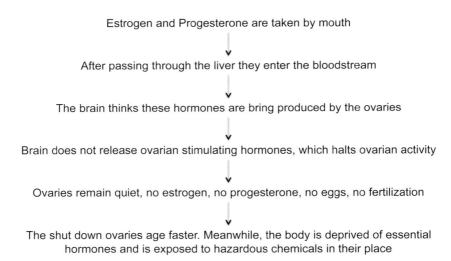

Estrogen and Progesterone are taken by mouth

↓

After passing through the liver they enter the bloodstream

↓

The brain thinks these hormones are bring produced by the ovaries

↓

Brain does not release ovarian stimulating hormones, which halts ovarian activity

↓

Ovaries remain quiet, no estrogen, no progesterone, no eggs, no fertilization

↓

The shut down ovaries age faster. Meanwhile, the body is deprived of essential hormones and is exposed to hazardous chemicals in their place

Birth control pills are made of hormone-like substances that do not occur naturally in the human body. These hormone-like substances are manufactured by the pharmaceutical industry and are often referred to as "synthetic."

Problems with Birth Control Pills

- Birth control pills have numerous harmful side effects, many of which are written in small print on the package insert. If these risks were not real or significant, manufacturers would not be required to declare them.

- The synthetic chemicals in birth control pills do not

perform identically to the body's own hormones. They are not broken down the same way, which makes them more potent because of uncontrolled signaling. A hormone that is not identical to what the body makes must be considered harmful until proven otherwise. (See Chapter 15, Different Types of Hormones: Natural, Bioidentical, Synthetic)

- Once non-bioidentical hormones are broken down (metabolized), their byproducts are potentially harmful and carcinogenic.

- Birth control pills are designed to mimic real hormones in the brain's hormone control system. They signal the brain to not release ovary-stimulating hormones (FSH, LH). Normal ovarian function is halted, while the body is exposed to hormone-like chemicals.

- Birth control pills enter the liver circulation before they enter the general circulation. A high dose of estrogen in the liver on a daily basis is not normal. The liver inappropriately makes proteins such as blood clotting proteins and C-reactive proteins (CRP), which have harmful long-term effects.

- Ovarian hormones are produced in a distinct rhythm, which has countless benefits to the whole body, including their interaction with other glands and hormones. Hormones in birth control pills are not provided in a natural rhythm.

Chapter 15

Different Types of Hormones:
Natural, Bioidentical, Synthetic

Natural Hormones

In order for a hormone to be labeled "natural," its source must exist somewhere in nature, either in plants or animals. Natural hormones are not created in a lab. This has nothing to do with safety of the hormone or what is natural to the human body.

For decades, natural hormones have been used to treat menopausal symptoms. These were not identical to what our bodies make, and had serious side effects.

For example, estrogens extracted from a pregnant horses' urine are natural, with benefits to the horse but not necessarily to a human female. These natural estrogens have been FDA approved, but are harmful.

Yams contain many steroid hormones with some components molecularly identical (bioidentical) to what a human female makes. The bioidentical hormones in the yams need to be extracted and purified in the lab.

The term "natural" is misleading as it is often mistaken for being synonymous with "safe." The estrogens in the pregnant horses' urine are natural, as is the thyroid hormone mix from a pig and growth hormone from a cadaver. Countless other harmful substances also occur in nature.

Bioidentical Hormones

Bioidentical means that the molecular structure is identical to what is naturally produced by the human body. Bioidentical hormones can be manufactured in a lab or extracted from nature; the source does not matter as long as the actual product is molecularly identical to what the body makes.

Molecular Integrity of Bioidentical Hormones

The correct molecular structure is critical. A change in an atom on a molecule changes the molecule's properties.

For example, the molecular structure of water is: H_2O (two hydrogen atoms and one oxygen atom). Hydrogen peroxide, which is not quite the same, has the molecular structure H_2O_2. The difference is only one extra oxygen atom.

Methanol is poisonous and has a molecular structure of CH_3OH. "Regular" alcohol is CH_3CH_2OH. A little difference can cause blindness and the difference between life and death.

As mentioned before, the difference between the molecular structure of estradiol and testosterone is one hydrogen (H) atom. There are more molecular differences in the structures of bioidentical hormones and their synthetic FDA approved versions in the market.

Limitations of Bioidentical Hormones

Bioidentical is a broad term. For example, the human ovary makes the estrogen type estradiol. A small amount of estrone is also made in the human ovary. Estriol is not made in the human ovary, but it exists in the blood after it is converted from estradiol. Therefore, although estradiol, estrone, and estriol are all bioidentical and coexist in the blood stream, the fact that they are bioidentical has nothing to do with how and if they should be replaced.

This simple concept needs to be understood. Hormones should be replaced as "bio-correctly" as possible.

Synthetic Hormones

If the molecular structure of a hormone is not identical to what is produced in the human body, it is referred to as synthetic.

Synthetic hormones come from a variety of sources. They can be created in the lab or extracted from natural sources such as plants and animals.

Synthetic hormones act on many of the same receptor sites as bioidentical hormones, thereby triggering a similar response in many areas of the body. However, the similarity is limited, as synthetic hormones have many unwanted and uncontrolled effects. For example, the body's own estrogen has beneficial effects on the cardiovascular system that are not paralleled with synthetic estrogen.[130]

Synthetic estrogens, also known as estrogenic products, have received a special class of warning from the FDA called a "black box" warning because of the risk of venous thrombosis (blood clots).[45]

Chapter 16

The Great Hormone Replacement Controversy

Early History

Prior to 2002, the topic of hormone replacement was relatively quiet. Throughout the world, women were given hormone replacement for relieving menopausal symptoms. Research articles were published from academic centers around the world showing the benefits of estrogen and progesterone.

There was never any consensus or standardization on any aspect of hormone uses other than that they were FDA approved. The benefits women were reporting (for example, reduction in hot flashes) were generally positive. However, many women could not tolerate the side effects of synthetic hormones.

Beginning of the Controversy

Based on decades of exhaustive research and studies, large research trials were developed. Two of the largest were the Women's Health Initiative (WHI) Study (initiated in 1991) and the Heart and Estrogen/Progesterone Replacement Study (HERS) (initiated in 1992).

The Women's Health Initiative Study

This study shook the world of postmenopausal hormone replacement, and the aftershocks are still being felt.

The study was heavily flawed, and not many physicians in the United States were intellectually equipped to question the study.

This landmark study, the largest of its kind, was funded by the National Institute of Health (NIH), and recruited thousands of women from about forty top U.S. clinical centers.

Because the study had been designed by the country's leading physicians from prestigious medical centers, it was routine for busy physicians to proudly rely on the data given.

The WHI Study Design

The study was designed to define the risks and benefits of interventions, including hormone therapy, to potentially prevent heart disease, breast and colorectal cancer, and osteoporotic fractures in postmenopausal women.[131]

The WHI study was divided into several parts including the effects of low-fat diet, and calcium and vitamin D supplements. But the part that became famous was the hormone replacement on postmenopausal women.

For the entire study, 373,092 women were screened, and about 161,809 were enrolled.

For the hormone replacement part of the WHI study about 27,347 women were enrolled.

WHI Study Hormone Components

The hormone part of the WHI study consisted of two components: Estrogen and progestin,[289] and estrogen only.[132]

For the first component (estrogen and progestin):

- A total of about 16,608 women were recruited.

- Ages ranged from fifty to seventy-nine.

- All participants had an intact uterus (i.e., had had no hysterectomy).

- About 8,506 women received 0.625 mg conjugated equine estrogen (derived from pregnant horses' urine) in pill form every day and 2.5 mg medroxyprogesterone acetate (synthetic progesterone) also in pill form every day.

- About 8,102 were given placebos (pills that looked like the hormones but were not).

- The planned duration for the study was eight and a half years. Monitoring began in fall 1997.

- The study was terminated in May 2002 (about three years prior to the projected completion) by the Data Safety Monitoring Board (DSMB) when a predetermined threshold of excess breast cancer was reached.[131]

- Overall results: Increase in coronary heart disease, invasive breast cancer, stroke, and pulmonary embolism (blood clot in the lung). Reduced risk in colorectal cancer, endometrial cancer, and hip fracture.

For the second component (estrogen only):

- A total of about 10,739 women were recruited.

- Ages ranged from fifty to seventy-nine.

- No participant had a uterus present (all women had previously undergone hysterectomy).

- Some women were given 0.625 mg conjugated equine estrogen (derived from pregnant horses' urine) in pill form every day.

- Some women were given a placebo.

- The planned duration for the study was about eight years.

- The study was terminated in March 2004 after almost seven years (about one year prior to the projected completion) by the NIH (the people who funded it) due to increased incidence of stroke and failure to prevent heart disease.

- Overall results: Risk of stroke increased, risk of hip fracture decreased. Neutral effect was seen on the incidence of coronary heart disease and breast cancer.

The aftermath of the study was equally disturbing. The presentation of the results from the first component was broadcast in medical training centers across the country. The dramatic intensity of the data presentation created an environment of intellectual unity that any existing or upcoming physician would seem a fool to question.

Results of the WHI Study

Physicians everywhere were given the guidelines that:

- Hormones should not be used for prevention of heart disease.

- Hormones can increase the risk of breast cancer, and should not be used for anyone with a history of breast cancer.

- If there is no personal or family history of breast cancer, women experiencing hot flashes and other disturbing symptoms of menopause can be given the smallest dose of hormones for the shortest possible time. However, antidepressants could also be offered.

- If there is a family or personal history of breast cancer, hormones are contraindicated. Suitable alternative treatments are antidepressants.

As a result, many women started taking antidepressants. Some stubbornly continued the hormones due to intolerable side effects of menopause. Others went to the Internet to find yet other solutions.

Meanwhile, Around the World ...

The prestigious *British Medical Journal* (BMJ) and countless other medical authorities including physicians within the United States were horrified with the disturbing level of medical ignorance and mismanagement.

It was a difficult task to oppose and question the work of the WHI team. This was a team of formidable, united, powerful individuals who made it almost impossible to clarify the misinformation they provided.

As suggested by a clinical professor from Emory University School of Medicine, the presentation made by the WHI authors in July 2002 changed with each new publication from the group, undermining the credibility of the research and of the medical community as a whole.[131]

Critical points were raised and need to be understood:

- This study did not use hormones that are identical to those made by the human body. Therefore, this issue was not *hormone* replacement but replacement with hormone-like chemicals—in women who were already aging and ailing.

- Of special note, the progesterone analogue was a chemically modified version of progesterone (medroxyprogesterone acetate) on which numerous articles have been published in the medical literature explaining its significant detrimental effects on the human body.[7,112] (See Chapter 17, Progesterone).

- The study did not consider that ovarian hormones are produced in a rhythm. If ovarian hormones are to be replaced, the rhythm is critical for balanced health.

- Not giving progesterone to women without a uterus was a baffling medical decision. Progesterone is needed for the breast, brain, and everywhere else estrogen goes. Providing over 5000 women with estrogen without progesterone was a very disappointing decision.

- The fact that these women had no uterus should have begged the question, why? Perhaps they had been naturally imbalanced for years on too much estrogen without progesterone leading to uterine fibroids and other issues.

- Estrogen without progesterone is a setup for trouble; furthermore, estrogen in the form of Premarin® is categorically wrong. It promotes inflammation, blood clots and breast cancer due to its oral (by mouth) entry, as well as containing estrogens the human body does not make.

- Many reputable studies have shown that estrogen by mouth is a problem.[133,134] The liver responds to oral estrogen by making proteins including ones that increase blood clots and inflammation. Why the study ignored such critical data has still not been explained.

The WHI study was, without doubt, a failure. But, the damage is continuously being felt due to the way the study has been repeatedly misinterpreted and covered up. Because the truth has not been acknowledged, and because information has been covered up, millions of women suffered and continue to suffer by making wrong ill-informed choices.

The confusion stemming from the WHI study needs to be clarified. It does not matter how the results are interpreted; the study was wrong by design.

There is a lot to be learned about hormones, but, until we have the answers we need, it is important to work within the knowledge we have.

The Heart and Estrogen/Progestin Replacement Study (HERS)

The Heart and Estrogen/Progestin Replacement Study (HERS) was another large study that very significantly confused physicians and their patients. There was an initial HER study (HERS), and later the HERS II, which was a follow-up.

- 2,763 women participated in HERS; 2,321 of these went on to participate in the HERS II.

- The study was designed to primarily measure nonfatal myocardial infarction (heart attack) and death from coronary heart disease (CHD).

- Secondary   factors   measured   were   coronary

revascularization, hospitalization for unstable angina or congestive heart failure, nonfatal ventricular arrhythmia, sudden death, stroke or transient ischemic attack, and peripheral arterial disease.

- Results: There were no significant decreases in rates of primary CHD events or secondary cardiovascular events among women assigned to the hormone group compared to those assigned to the placebo group in HERS or HERS II, or overall.[135]

- Conclusions:[135,136,137] Many conclusions were derived but they all were confusing.

- Fact: the HERS, like the WHI study, used synthetic hormones.

Several other major studies, including the Postmenopausal Estrogen/Progestin Interventions (PEPI) trial,[138] demonstrated the benefits of hormone replacement without significant adverse outcome. They also used synthetic hormones.

Chapter 17
Breast and Ovarian Cancer

Breast Cancer

The topic of breast cancer is very complex, and beyond the scope of this book. Dr. Khalid Mahmud in his book, *Keeping aBreast: Ways to Stop Breast Cancer,*[296] has explained this topic in detail with medical references.

Many studies have looked at the effects of synthetic estrogen and progesterone on the risk of breast cancer; however, studies to evaluate the risk of breast cancer with replacement of bioidentical hormones are still lacking.

Although the WHI study showed a slight increase of breast cancer in women on synthetic estrogen and synthetic progesterone, there was no increased incidence in the women on estrogen alone, pointing to medroxyprogesterone acetate (MPA) as the culprit.

In a study done in 1999, 319 women with a history of breast cancer were placed on estrogen replacement therapy and evaluated for new or recurrent cases. The study showed a decreased incidence in women on estrogen replacement therapy.[115] Other studies have also reported no increase in breast cancer in women on estrogen therapy.[139,140]

Many studies have looked into the different factors that could contribute to the incidence of breast cancer.[288,298] Other than genetic factors, there is strong belief that a greater lifetime exposure to estrogen without progesterone balance leads to a greater risk of breast cancer. It has been stated in numerous medical publications that early menarche (age at which a period starts) and late menopause (cessation of periods) is a risk factor for breast cancer, as are having no pregnancies and not breast feeding.[141,142,294]

Of note is that, during the first few years of the menstrual history (after menarche) as well as during the last few years (perimenopause), there are many anovulatory cycles during which estrogen is present without progesterone. This is a known risk for breast cancer.

However, some important points need to be considered when making a decision:

- No study to date has proved or showed that bioidentical hormone replacement can cause breast cancer or increase the risk.

- Any study done to date, including the WHI study, that shows negative effects of hormones on the breast have been poorly designed with hormone-like substances which should not have been used in the first place.

- Many studies demonstrate that oral estrogen causes more breast cancer risk than transdermal (through the skin) estrogen.[143]

- A woman makes the most estrogen in her youth. In pregnancy, a woman's estrogen level is far higher than at any other time; yet the risk of breast cancer is the least during youth and pregnancy.[144] It has been noted that, if a woman gets breast cancer during pregnancy, which is an extremely rare situation, the cancer is very aggressive. The hormone makeup in pregnancy is specific and is never reproduced at any other time in life.

- Most cases of breast cancer occur after menopause. Typically there have been several years of anovulatory cycles (menstrual cycles without ovulation), which create an absence of progesterone balance in the second half of the cycle.

- It is generally considered that there are two times in a woman's life when she is exposed to estrogen without progesterone protection. The first is the beginning of menses; the second is perimenopause. It is thought that the duration of these "estrogen only" years determines the risk of breast cancer.[144]

- Many women with breast cancer have lacked progesterone balance for years. If there is a family history of breast cancer, ovarian function needs to be evaluated. At minimum, progesterone and estrogen should be measured on day twenty-one of the menstrual cycle (if there is a cycle) and estrogen on day ten or eleven. If it is seen that progesterone is low compared to the estrogen, it would be breast protective to correctly replace progesterone.

Ovarian Cancer

The data on the effects of bioidentical hormone replacement on ovarian cancer is virtually non-existent. Also, there have been no studies to show what happens if ovarian hormones are replaced in the ovarian pattern.

One of the largest collections of data has been from a Danish study recently published in the *Journal of the American Medical Association* (JAMA). The study concluded that, regardless of duration of use, formulation, estrogen dose, regimen, progestin type, and route of administration, hormone therapy was associated with an increased risk of ovarian cancer. The risk was approximated at one extra ovarian cancer for roughly 8,300 women taking hormone therapy each year.[145]

Ovarian cancer is one of the most feared cancers in women. It is usually detected after it has spread, at which time the treatment has limited success. However, the Danish study did not evaluate bioidentical hormones administered topically in a natural ovarian rhythm. The ovaries are very sensitive to correct signaling from the entire body including the brain. Giving exogenous (from outside the body) hormones in an unnatural way has unknown and unpredictable consequences.

A study published in 2002 stated that women on estrogen alone, particularly for an extended time, were at a greater risk for ovarian cancer. The same risk was not seen with estrogen and (synthetic) progesterone.[247] However, it is disturbing that women were given estrogen without progesterone at all.

Chapter 18

Treatment with Ovarian Hormones

(Estrogen and Progesterone)

When replacement of ovarian hormones is considered, some crucial points need to be considered:

- The route that estradiol (estrogen) is administered

- The correct molecular form of the hormones is given. (i.e., bioidentical)

- The dosing and rhythm is as close to the ovarian rhythm as possible

Route of administration: Oral versus Topical

Although the medical literature does not describe the implications of oral versus transdermal (topical) progesterone very well, there is plenty of data to demonstrate how oral estrogen is detrimental to health. When estrogen in any molecular form, including the bioidentical estradiol, is taken by mouth, there is a significant response by the liver:

- The liver is a vital organ whose main functions include detoxification and protein synthesis.

- Once anything (other than fat) is taken by mouth and passes the stomach, it goes to the liver for detoxification and "evaluation" before reaching the general circulation.

- Nature has designed estrogen to reach the liver in distinct doses from the ovaries through the general circulation. There are specific times the liver "sees" high doses of estrogen, and is designed to respond; for example, in pregnancy and once a month during the menstrual cycle

- As a response to high doses of estrogen, the liver increases its production of special proteins, which promote blood clotting (hypercoagulation) and inflammation.[146,147,148,149,150,151,152,153] On the right occasion, this is a good thing and the body can sustain it; however, it is not a good thing on a daily basis as is the case with oral estrogen for hormone replacement.

When a hormone is applied to the skin, it goes from:

Skin
↓
Fat
↓
General circulation
↓
Liver

(Normal concentration, as it is diluted in the blood before going to the liver)

When a hormone is taken by mouth, it goes from:

Mouth
↓
Stomach
↓
Small intestines
↓
Liver

(High concentration as it is not entered the general circulation yet)
↓
General circulation
(Normal concentration)

Also, of note, is, if a woman has growth hormone deficiency, taking oral estrogen makes the deficiency worse. Studies show that oral estrogen affects the growth hormone effects on the liver by decreasing insulin-like growth factor (IGF-I levels). This is not seen in topical administration.[154]

Correct Form of Hormone

The medical community is getting close to the consensus that bioidentical hormone replacement is safer than synthetic hormone replacement.

Some difficulties with bioidentical hormones are:

- Bioidentical hormones cannot be patented because they exist naturally in the human body. Without the financial incentives of a patentable product it is not lucrative for any single company to pay millions of dollars for an FDA approval.

- Bioidentical hormones can be made by any licensed compounding pharmacy, which leads to a lack of standardization.

- Bioidentical hormones are not part of the medical curriculum, and physicians are not trained to treat hormones deficiencies that do not cause disease.

- Bioidentical hormones are not "standard of care," where synthetic ones are. The fear of malpractice law suits has led physicians to do only that which will protect them in court, which today is only standard-of-care medicine.

Dosing and Rhythm

As mentioned earlier, hormones are cell signals. There is no known hormone that is made and released in a constant dose. Estradiol and progesterone are two ovarian hormones that have a very distinct pattern of production.

We have known the ovarian hormone pattern for centuries; it is clearly defined in every medical, endocrinology, and gynecology text book.

The European physicians practicing hormone replacement recognized that giving a linear dose (same dose every day) led to cell resistance, and the hormones did not work well. To overcome this problem, they recommended taking a week off per month so the cells could have time to "readjust." The exact mechanism was not known, but this was based on the understanding that there is some pattern and the hormones become ineffective if given continuously, day in day out.

A similar concept is seen in type II diabetes where years of sustained carbohydrate intake leads to constant insulin release by the pancreas, causing cell receptors not to recognize insulin effectively (insulin resistance).

The dose-dependent effect of estrogen has been widely studied.[155] For example; estrogen stimulates the liver to produce many different types of proteins that are needed for different functions. The types and quantities of these proteins are dependent on the dose of estrogen the liver is exposed to.

Significance of the Ovarian Cycle

Although estrogen and progesterone are dose-dependent hormones, they certainly have shown some benefits at low doses. However, giving the body hormones for a long time in doses and patterns that it is not genetically recognized to receive is a health risk.

Estrogen cycles regularly and predictably every month. At its peak, it initiates a chain of events that causes its own temporary shutdown, triggers ovulation, increases testosterone production, while having instructed the production of receptors for other hormones.

To get the full benefit of ovarian estrogen (estradiol), it should be dosed as closely to the ovarian cycle as possible. The extent to which estrogen binds and therefore signals an event is influenced by which type of estrogen it is and what its concentration is.[144]

During the first half of the ovarian cycle (follicular phase) estrogen up regulates (makes more of) its own receptors as well as progesterone receptors.[103] Progesterone has an opposite effect, it down regulates its own as well as estrogen receptors.[144]

If there are no receptors for the hormone, the hormone cannot fully perform its job. This is yet another reason not to give progesterone the entire month.

There is a lot to be understood about the dose-dependent effects of estrogen. We know that healthy women before menopause produce estrogen in a specific pattern. This rhythm of fertility keeps the entire brain and body in an optimum state of health for supporting reproduction. The menstrual bleeding is not the only reason we need to cycle hormones.

Nondiscriminatory Estrogen Effects

There are some effects of estrogen that are less discriminating to the type of estrogen, its dose, or rhythm.

Hot flashes

- A woman has hot flashes at low levels of estrogen. There is no fixed level of estrogen at which hot flashes occur, and each woman's experience is different.

- Hot flashes do not last forever. When the estrogen dips very low, for example, in late fifties onwards, it is rare to have hot flashes.

- No one really knows what the mechanisms of hot flashes are, although there are many speculations. We do know that they are relieved by estrogen replacement, even if it's replaced without a rhythm.

- Progesterone and serotonin-increasing antidepressants can reduce hot flashes to some extent.

- We know that estrogen has direct effect on serotonin receptors. It is hypothesized that serotonin activity is involved in temperature regulation. This is the basis on which antidepressants such as selective serotonin reuptake inhibitors (SSRIs) and Tricyclic antidepressants are given to relieve hot flashes. However, altering brain neurotransmitters without a thorough understanding of the complex network of events, a measurable goal, or understanding long-term implications is an unconscionable act of medicine, especially when safer alternatives are present.

Osteoporosis

- From the studies such as the WHI study and HERS, it was seen that osteoporosis, measured by decrease in bone fractures, was reduced with hormone replacement.

- Both these studies used low, constant (static) doses of estrogens as well as synthetic progesterone.

Urogenital Function

- Estriol, which is irreversibly produced from estradiol and estrone, is known to improve the functioning of the urogenital tract.

- Local administration of estriol has been known to stimulate function of the urinary tract and genital tissue.

In Summary

- Any hormone replaced—especially steroid hormones such as estrogen and progesterone—should only be bioidentical, which means that it is molecularly identical to what the human body makes. To deviate from this is a health risk. Synthetic hormones, not identical to what the body makes, act in unpredictable ways, and should be considered harmful until proven otherwise.

- Estrogen should never be given by mouth on regular basis. The liver reacts by producing excessive proteins that could be harmful. Controlled release with topical application has the advantage of avoiding the initial liver exposure by first dispersing into the general blood circulation.

- In replacing ovarian hormones, the ovarian rhythm should be followed. Any other dosing schedule has unpredictable consequences. Although constant, linear dosing may have some benefits, the optimum benefits cannot be reached unless nature's pattern is observed.

T.S. Wiley and the Wiley Protocol®

T. S. Wiley is the author of *Sex, Lies, and Menopause: The Shocking Truth About Synthetic Hormones and the benefits of Natural Alternatives,* along with, Julie Taguchi, and Bent Formby. She is also author of *Lights Out: Sleep, Sugar, and Survival* along with Bent Formby. Although, T. S. Wiley has no formal education in medicine, her understanding and work in the field of hormone replacement is remarkable.

While anti-aging physicians around the world were developing the science of bioidentical hormone replacement, and traditional medicine was ignoring it completely, T.S. Wiley independently studied the medical literature to understand how hormones affect our health.

T. S. Wiley's basic conclusions were:

- Hormones need to be replaced

- Hormones must be bioidentical

- Hormones should be applied topically

- Hormones should be administered in the natural rhythm

The timing of the publication of these findings was interesting because several parallel, independent events were occurring:

- The nation's top medical centers were involved in studies such as the WHI study and HERS. Synthetic hormones were still being used in a constant, linear dose and mainly orally.

- Anti-aging physicians around the world were treating menopausal symptoms with bioidentical hormones. Topical rather than oral hormones were being used. For the estrogen component some of these physicians were giving *Biest* (a combination of estradiol (E2) and estriol (E3)), while others were giving *Triest* (a combination of estrone (E1), estradiol (E2), and estriol (E3)). All were giving bioidentical progesterone.

- Most U.S. anti-aging physicians were following the European protocol of giving a few days off per month of estrogen and or progesterone, recognizing that hormones need some "time off." As mentioned earlier, there was no consensus in dosing patterns.

- T.S. Wiley was the only person recommending hormone replacement in the ovarian rhythm, with bioidentical hormones, specifically estradiol and progesterone.

Wiley recognized that hormones should be applied *topically* to avoid the unwanted liver response. She also realized that estradiol is the only estrogen that should be replaced, as it is what the ovaries predominantly make. But, Wiley's simple and most profound observation was that ovarian hormones should only be replaced in the *ovarian rhythm.*

Physicians in top medical centers still question hormone replacement without reflecting on simple scientific principles. It is not that these physicians are not capable of understanding the medical literature; the strong political environment of the medical system takes away the freedom of thinking and practicing real medicine.

Informed Choice

Women have the right to choose what they do about hormone replacement. But a woman's choice should be as informed as possible. It is important to gain knowledge—while paying attention to the source of the information.

Chapter 19

Testosterone in Women

Women and men both produce testosterone; however, it is *not* the major sex steroid hormone in normal, fertile women. Testosterone is dose related and has different effects in men and women. Testosterone has many functions in healthy women. The exact rhythm of testosterone production in women is not as clearly understood as the estradiol and progesterone rhythm.

How, Where, and When do Women Make Testosterone?

The major portion of testosterone in women is made from the conversion of DHEA and androstenedione (from the adrenal glands) outside the adrenal glands. It is also made in the ovaries where it is mostly converted to estradiol before it enters the general circulation.

- Fertile women produce more testosterone around ovulation. This peak in testosterone is nature's design to increase libido, enhancing the chance of conception.

- It is still not clear if this mid-cycle testosterone peak comes from the ovaries or the adrenal precursors (DHEA and androstenedione), or both.

- After menopause and decline in ovarian function, a woman's testosterone comes from the conversion of adrenal hormones (DHEA, androstenedione). The pattern of production is not understood, nor do we understand the brain's exact role.

- Menopause is also associated with an increasing testosterone/estrogen ratio. It is commonly observed that women with healthy adrenal glands become slightly more masculine. For example, there can be slight coarsening of facial features, a change in fat distribution, chin hair, oily skin, and voice changes.

- Healthy, fertile women do not make testosterone the entire month, certainly not in a constant dose. The long-term consequences of giving continuous-dose testosterone to a woman to restore libido are not known.[156,157]

Abnormal Testosterone Levels in Women

- Some studies suggest that relatively high amount of testosterone and estrogens are associated with endometrial cancer.[158] More studies are needed in this area. However, because testosterone is converted to estrogen, it is important to ensure that there is adequate balance of progesterone in the system.

- If a woman has healthy adrenal glands, it makes no sense to replace testosterone to restore libido, especially before restoring the youthful estrogen/progesterone rhythm.

- If a woman's adrenal glands are not functioning well, it is much more important to evaluate and treat that problem before worrying about the libido.

- Many women will testify to feeling great on testosterone, but of note is that almost any steroid hormone given will initially feel good. The long-term consequences of unnatural dosing are unknown at this time.[159]

- Although limited studies have been done on the benefits of testosterone on menopausal women, several studies indicate that the improvement in protein synthesis and muscle strength seen in them is insignificant.[160]

- However, testosterone is dose related, and it is clinically seen that body builders who take unprescribed testosterone (purchased over the Internet) see an improvement in muscle mass. Again, the safety of doing this is unknown and will likely never be studied due to the possible harmful effects.

- Women with polycystic ovary syndrome have high circulating levels of testosterone. As mentioned in Chapter 13, Polycystic Ovary Syndrome, medical consequences of high testosterone are unfavorable and linked to the undesired metabolic syndrome,[128,129,161] which also is linked to too little testosterone in men.[162]

Testosterone Replacement in Women

There are very few circumstances for which a woman should be supplemented with testosterone. If the adrenal glands are healthy, then correct dosing and cycling of the ovarian hormones estradiol and progesterone should allow the appropriate testosterone release. If the adrenals are not healthy, then testosterone/libido is of a lesser initial concern than identifying and correcting the adrenal problem.

Testosterone-estrogen Pellets

This is a new practice adopted by many anti-aging physicians, and is heavily marketed. Testosterone plus estrogen in pellet form are placed under the skin in the gluteal region. The pellets are designed to slowly "dissolve," and disappear over the course of several months.

- There is no hormonal rhythm with this method.

- Initially, due to such high doses of testosterone, women feel great. This begins to change over the next few months when the testosterone is invariably at a higher ratio in the blood than estrogen while both are declining.

- The pellets cannot be removed.

- Progesterone is not given in the pellets (which is a good thing). But, estrogen should always be replaced with progesterone. However, it would be challenging to appropriately replace progesterone while estrogen has no rhythm other than a constant decline.

Chapter 20

Testosterone in Men

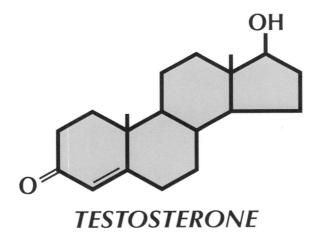

TESTOSTERONE

Testosterone is the major sex hormone in men and is primarily made in the testes. A small amount is also made from the adrenal gland hormones DHEA and androstenedione.

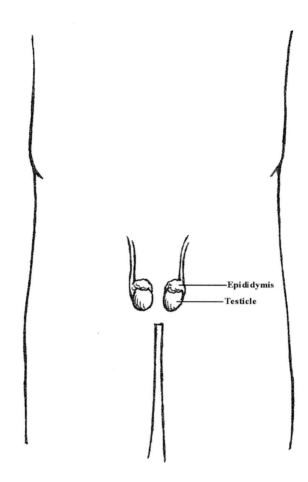

Like all steroid hormones, testosterone is also made from cholesterol.

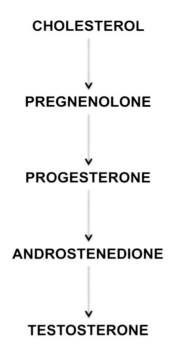

CHOLESTEROL

v

PREGNENOLONE

v

PROGESTERONE

v

ANDROSTENEDIONE

v

TESTOSTERONE

Fate of Testosterone

- Some of the testosterone in the testes is converted to estradiol within the testes and is thought to help in sperm development.

- A certain amount of testosterone is converted to estrogen outside the testes in several places. The estrogen converted from testosterone has many important functions for men.[163]

- Testosterone is also converted to dihydrotestosterone (DHT), which is thought to be a more potent androgen.

DHT cannot be converted to estrogen as testosterone can.

- Testosterone circulates in the blood mostly bound to special proteins made in the liver. About 60 percent of circulating testosterone is bound to sex hormone-binding globulin (SHBG), 38 percent is bound to albumin, and about 2 percent remain "free".[164]

- Of the gonadal hormones, testosterone production is by far the greatest. Per day there is approximately fifty to one hundred times less DHT production and approximately three to five hundred times less estrogen production.[164]

Declining Testosterone

Testosterone in aging men declines gradually and progressively. The changes seen in aging men such as muscle and bone weakness, increased fat mass, and reduced sexual function among many are also seen in young men who have documented testosterone deficiency.[165]

Several studies have shown that elderly men with low serum testosterone and estradiol have the highest risk of mortality.[166,167]

Indirect Testosterone Effects

Many of testosterone's important functions occur when testosterone acts directly on the cells. Other functions are indirect and occur when testosterone at some point converts to estrogen and DHT. For example, many of the critical functions of testosterone do not occur until it converts to estradiol and acts on the brain, bones, and facilitates lipid metabolism.[168]

For the body to function optimally there has to be a correct ratio, balance, and rhythm of the various hormones.

Dose Effect

The effects of testosterone are dose dependant.[169] Not only does testosterone have its own particular dose-dependent effects, but at different circulating levels it converts to estrogen and DHT.

Actions of Testosterone, DHT, and Estrogen

Testosterone plays a critical role in the healthy functioning of the human body, especially in men, where it the major sex steroid.

Brain

- Testosterone has multiple beneficial effects on the brain, directly and indirectly. It has been demonstrated that testosterone improves cognition, including visual-spatial skills in patients with mild to moderate Alzheimer's disease.[170]

- There are studies that link testosterone imbalance to cluster headaches.[171]

- Giving testosterone to men with testosterone deficiency has been demonstrated to improve mood.[174] The effects appear to be dose related.[169]

Cardiovascular

- Testosterone has been shown to cause coronary artery dilation and increase blood flow in men with established coronary artery disease.[175]

- The estrogen converted from testosterone is also known to have protective effects on the blood vessel walls and prevent heart disease.[176] In older men, lower total testosterone levels have been associated with higher incidence of stroke and transient ischemic attacks (TIA or "mini strokes") .[177]

Growth Hormone

There is abundant medical literature on the effects of testosterone on growth hormone release. This may be partly due to the direct effects of testosterone on the brain's growth hormone releasing axis, and partly indirectly due to estrogen.[178]

Insulin Sensitivity and the Metabolic Syndrome

- Metabolic syndrome, (a combination of disorders, including insulin resistance, abnormal lipid profile, high blood pressure, excess fat and increased chances for cardiovascular disease) a leading cause of mortality in aging men, has consistently been shown to improve with testosterone replacement.[180] However, it is important to understand that testosterone is dose dependant, and too much can have adverse effects.

- Studies support that testosterone has a positive effect on insulin sensitivity, and insulin resistance.[161,180] It is thought that testosterone suppresses the fat cells from producing a substance called adiponectin, which causes insulin resistance.[181] However, it seems that in women who produce too much testosterone, as is the case with polycystic ovary syndrome, the low adiponectin from too much testosterone does not have this beneficial effect on insulin resistance.[161]

Lipid Profile

- Testosterone is documented to have beneficial effects on the lipid profile. Studies show that testosterone lowers the atherogenic component of LDL (the oxidized portion), without altering the HDL.[183]

- The mechanism has not been established; however, it is speculated that testosterone improves the structure of cell membranes and facilitates LDL receptor production and function, so that cholesterol can enter the cells and be utilized.

Musculoskeletal

- Studies show that men with rheumatoid arthritis have a

higher frequency of hypogonadism (low testosterone).[184]

- Studies have demonstrated that high normal levels of testosterone and DHEA predict a greater than 60 percent reduction in falls in both older men and women.[185]

- Testosterone has long been known to build muscle mass. There is a profound effect at puberty when boys gain greater than 30 percent more muscle mass than girls.[100]

- Some studies have shown that testosterone favorably redistributes fat and muscle in men over sixty-five;[186] however, other studies are not as conclusive.[159]

- The muscle mass building effects of testosterone have led to the abuse of testosterone and its precursor androstenedione ("andro"), which is illegally available over the internet.

- Studies show that testosterone supplementation along with exercise may be an important strategy for maintaining quality of life in elderly men.[187]

Sexual Function

- Testosterone has long been associated with libido. Testosterone deficiency is also closely linked to erectile dysfunction.[172,173,188,189] Testosterone is needed for the growth and function of the penile nerves and tissue.[172] Results of several studies have suggested that testosterone therapy may be a valuable option in the treatment of erectile dysfunction.[190]

- Exogenous (externally given) testosterone has an effect of suppressing spermatogenesis and is being evaluated for male contraceptive.[191] This should not be confused with erectile function, which has a different mechanism. The concentration of testosterone in the testes needs to be at least one hundred times greater than blood levels for sperm development. When testosterone is replaced, the testes stop making their own testosterone, therefore sperm count plummets.

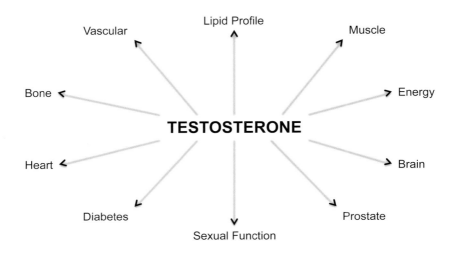

The Importance of Testosterone's Conversion to Estrogen

Some of the critical functions of testosterone occur after it is converted to estrogen by the enzyme aromatase:

- The brain and bones in both men and women need estrogen.

- Men have a higher ratio of estrogen to testosterone as they age. It appears that, as they age, their aromatase activity (testosterone to estrogen conversion) is protected.

- It is likely that sufficient testosterone is converted to estrogen to be used in critical areas such as the brain and bone before it is available for less-life-sustaining uses. (More studies are needed to clarify this.)

- If an aging man has a higher ratio of estrogen to testosterone, it is advisable to increase testosterone rather than block the conversion of testosterone to the much-needed estrogen.

Conversion to Dihydrotestosterone (DHT)

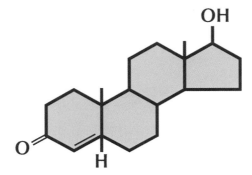

DHT - DIHYDROTESTOSTERONE

Dihydrotestosterone (DHT) is the most potent form of testosterone. Men generally have a higher ratio of DHT to testosterone as they age.

Certain medications used to treat benign prostatic hypertrophy (BPH) block the conversion of testosterone to DHT.

More research is needed to better understand the dose-dependent effect of testosterone.

Laboratory Measurement of Testosterone

Testosterone circulates freely in the blood; it also binds to special proteins. At minimum, free and total testosterone should be measured.

Older men have higher levels of total testosterone compared to free testosterone because the liver makes more testosterone-binding proteins.[192]

Timing

Testosterone levels are the highest in the morning, which is when they should be measured.

If a man is taking supplemental testosterone in a rhythm, the measurement should be taken on the days when the blood has the highest levels of testosterone.

Measuring Testosterone in Saliva, Urine, or Blood

We are still in the early years of measuring steroid hormones. There are limited studies that compare the accuracy of testing saliva, urine, and blood for the correct circulating levels of testosterone. However, a recent study comparing the reliability of blood versus saliva for measuring topically applied testosterone showed blood to be more reliable than saliva. The study concluded that, although saliva testing is appealing because it is noninvasive and less expensive, the routine use of saliva for measuring testosterone should not be supported.[193]

Studies also claim that measurement of salivary levels of steroid hormones (estrogen, progesterone, testosterone, DHEA, and aldosterone) are compromised because of the rapid fluctuations of steroid hormones in the saliva.[194]

Blood Testing

- The advantage of testing blood at this time is that it is the most reproducible and consistent method of measuring free and total testosterone.

- The limitation is that the blood levels do not always convey the complete picture. There are situations when blood levels are good but the patient is symptomatic due to various other reasons, including resistant cell receptors. Although this phenomenon usually resolves after a rhythm is given, much more needs to be understood.

Treatment with Testosterone in Men

Dosing

Although, it is clearly understood that testosterone is critical to well-being, the data on how to best administer testosterone is still not complete.

The testosterone rhythm is not as distinct or well understood as the ovarian estrogen and progesterone rhythm. Testosterone levels are highest in the morning and lowest at night; a monthly or seasonal rhythm may exist but is less understood.

Men who take testosterone on a constant schedule without a rhythm invariably get blunting of the beneficial effects after a few months, even if the blood levels look good. In these situations, taking a week off per month and perhaps a few days off in the middle of the month resets the cells to respond to testosterone better. This is a crude method, but works better than constant dosing.

Many men report beneficial results by injecting testosterone every four days with a dose skipped each month.

The Wiley Protocol® is based on placing men on a solar monthly cycle using topical testosterone cream, with dose elevations or decreases every four days. Again, the male testosterone rhythm is not completely understood.

Different Forms of Testosterone

Testosterone is available in many forms. The most common are oral, injectable, and topical.

- Oral testosterone is easy to take, but has unpredictable effects on blood levels and liver function. The testosterone in oil-based capsules enters blood through the lymph system, bypassing the liver and gives erratic blood levels.[195] Non-oil-based preparations of testosterone enter the liver circulation and may have damaging effects on the liver.[195]

- Injectable testosterone work well for those who are not averse to injecting themselves. Typically, injectable testosterone is administered biweekly, or every four days and skipping a dose per month.

- The daily pattern of testosterone—high in the morning and low at night—is necessary for optimal testosterone interaction with melatonin, thyroid hormone, growth hormone, as well as countless other molecules.[195] How the body adjusts to injecting testosterone every four days and skipping a dose per month is not understood, but men seem to respond very well to this method.

• Some studies show that topical application of cream- or gel-based testosterone allows the closest-to-natural blood levels.[195] However, the product needs to absorb adequately. Also, penetration of the gel or cream is variable between individuals. Gel-based testosterone has been popular because it penetrates the skin more easily than cream.

Importantly, how the patient feels is more of a predictor of adequate testosterone levels than lab values.[192]

Testicular Response

When testosterone is supplemented by any method, the testicular production of testosterone declines, as does the sperm count. This reduction in testicular function causes a reduction in testicular mass. Some practitioners suggest supplementing with additional hormones to stimulate testicular mass, but this treatment needs more studies and data. However, this phenomenon is being considered for male contraception.[191]

Chapter 21

The Prostate Gland and Cancer

The fact that testosterone replacement causes prostate cancer is a medical myth that was created many years ago; it has been nullified by several studies.[172]

There are no studies that demonstrate that testosterone supplements cause prostate cancer. Rather, it is seen that men get prostate cancer well into andropause when they have been testosterone deficient for years.

Numerous studies have been performed in which supplemental testosterone has been given to older men. There is no credible evidence that shows that testosterone replacement causes an increase in prostate size, an increase in prostate-specific antigen levels, or an increase in the number of prostate cancer cases.[196]

Studies have demonstrated that replacing testosterone in men who have low levels does not increase their incidence of prostate cancer beyond the incidence in the normal population.[197]

Studies have also demonstrated that patients with castration-resistant metastatic prostate cancer could safely be treated with high doses of testosterone.[198]

BPH (Benign prostatic hypertrophy) is a condition in aging men in which the prostate gland enlarges. BPH commonly follows diminishing levels of testosterone with normal aging. Testosterone is responsible for maintaining the strong wall of the prostate gland, thus preventing it from expanding. Estrogen is thought to maintain the inner part of the gland. The upset balance of testosterone and estrogen which occurs with aging, allows the prostate gland to increase in size. The annoyance associated with this condition is frequent urination with a slow, "dribbling" stream, resulting from the enlarged prostate gland pushing against the urinary system, interfering with the urine flow.

Chapter 22

Adrenal Glands

There are two adrenal glands; they are located above the kidneys.

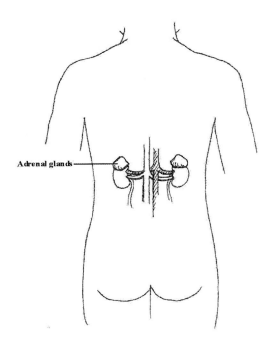

Adrenal glands

Hormones Produced in the Adrenal Glands

The hormones of the adrenal glands are essential for sustaining life, regulating metabolism, and adaptation to stress.

Disorders of the adrenal glands lead to numerous endocrine

diseases such as Cushing's syndrome, Addison's disease, hyperaldosteronism, polycystic ovarian syndrome, hirsutism, virilization, and many others including congenital diseases (birth disorders).

Adrenal Gland Structure

There are two distinct sections of the adrenal glands:

ADRENAL GLAND

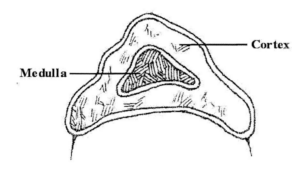

The inner part is called the medulla and produces catecholamines, which include:

- Norepinephrine

- Epinephrine

The outer part is called the cortex and produces steroid hormones, which include:

- Mineral corticoids, the main one of which is called aldosterone. Its main job is to regulate salt and water balance via the kidneys.

- Cortisol, which has numerous life sustaining functions,

and is the main hormone of stress, inflammation control, and immune suppression.

- Adrenal androgens, which consist of DHEA, DHEAS, and androstenedione. They are converted outside the adrenal glands to other androgens such as testosterone, DHT and estrogens.

Adrenal hormones communicate with each other, the brain chemicals (neurotransmitters), as well as hormones from other glands.

Catecholamines (Adrenalin)

The catecholamines norepinephrine and epinephrine are produced in the inner part of the adrenal glands. They are extremely fast acting and potent chemicals.

Although they are categorized as hormones, catecholamines also act as neurotransmitters. Neurotransmitters facilitate communication through nerve endings.

Norepinephrine is made primarily in nerve tissues, and only about 30 percent comes from the adrenal glands.

Epinephrine is made almost exclusively in the adrenal glands through the modification of norepinephrine.

Function of Catecholamines

Catecholamines have countless functions, but are mostly known for allowing us to perform beyond our normal capacity in the face of danger. When our heart "jumps" in the instance of fear:

- The brain sends a signal to the adrenal glands.

- Adrenalin (catecholamines) is released into the blood and reaches the heart.

- The heart beats faster.

All of this happens in the time frame of a heartbeat. Catecholamines increase blood glucose levels, increase heart rate and cardiac output while controlling blood flow in different organs facilitating the "fight or flight" response.

The following graphic illustrates the steps in the formation of adrenal catecholamines:

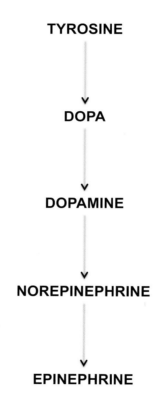

TYROSINE

DOPA

DOPAMINE

NOREPINEPHRINE

EPINEPHRINE

Adrenal Steroid Hormones

The cells of the cortex of the adrenal glands have numerous receptors for cholesterol. After cholesterol enters the cells, it converts to pregnenolone within the mitochondria, and then goes back into the main cell compartment to convert to other hormones.

There are three fates of pregnenolone in the adrenal gland:

In the middle cortex:

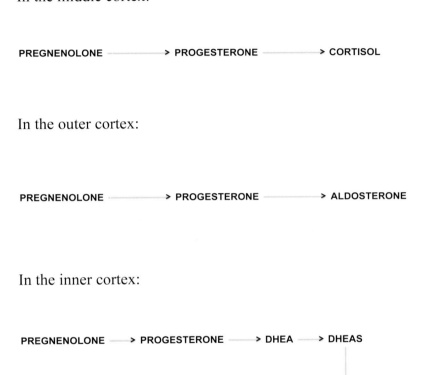

PREGNENOLONE ———> PROGESTERONE ———> CORTISOL

In the outer cortex:

PREGNENOLONE ———> PROGESTERONE ———> ALDOSTERONE

In the inner cortex:

PREGNENOLONE ——> PROGESTERONE ——> DHEA ——> DHEAS

ANDROSTENDIONE

Steroid hormones in the adrenal glands are regulated in a highly complex process involving the brain hormones corticotropin-releasing hormone (CRH) and adrenocorticotropic hormone (ACTH) as well as multiple other factors, which are less clearly understood.

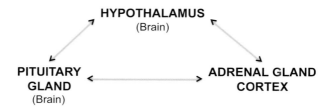

The brain produces hormones in a pulsatile manner, with daily, monthly, and seasonal rhythms. The rhythm and pulsatility is passed on to the glands they act upon.

- The hypothalamus in the brain makes CRH, which stimulates the pituitary gland in the brain to produce ACTH.

- ACTH acts on the adrenal glands to stimulate production of cortisol and all other adrenal steroids (other than aldosterone).

- Due to the pulsatility of CRH, ACTH also has pulsatility.

- ACTH is produced in higher quantities when cortisol is low due to negative feedback (i.e. the **deficiency** of one hormone signals the release of another).

Many other factors affect adrenal steroid synthesis but are less clearly understood.

Adrenal Androgens

Adrenarche is a developmental landmark of the adrenal glands, manifested by the growth of axillary and pubic hair. In young girls, adrenarche occurs several years before menarche (the first menstrual period). In males, adrenarche typically occurs a few years later than in females. It is very typical to see personality changes in both genders at this time.

The main adrenal androgens are:

- Dehydroepiandrosterone (DHEA) and dehydroepiandrosterone sulfate (DHEAS)

- Androstenedione

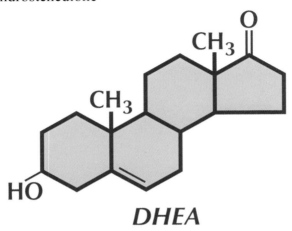

DHEA

Testosterone is produced from androstenedione and DHEA in tissues outside the adrenal glands.

Facts about DHEA and DHEAS:

- DHEA is made in the inner cortex of the adrenal glands. Once made, it is quickly broken down within about fifteen to thirty minutes; however, it is also converted to DHEAS (a sulfur group is added).

- It is not clearly understood what events cause DHEA to convert to DHEAS and vice versa.

- DHEAS has a longer half life than DHEA (it lasts seven to ten hours).[199]

- DHEAS can be converted back to DHEA outside of the adrenal gland.

- Once it leaves the adrenal glands, DHEA can also convert to testosterone and dihydrotestosterone DHT (a potent form of testosterone).

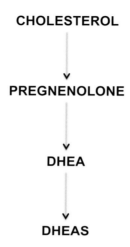

CHOLESTEROL

PREGNENOLONE

DHEA

DHEAS

DHEA is the main adrenal androgen. It is thought to be involved in estrogen synthesis in the fetus from the mother. In women, it is a major source for androgen synthesis. It becomes detectable in the blood at about age six. Within the next few years, the body responds with physical signs such as axillary and pubic hair growth, sweat gland maturation, and other signs of puberty. It is the main adrenal steroid responsible for adrenarche.

The levels of DHEA and DHEAS steadily peak until the mid-twenties and then start to decline with aging.[200] There is a linear decline of DHEA in both men and women by about 2 percent per year starting at about age 30.[201] The adrenal androgen decline seems to be more prominent in women than in men, and is thought to be due to the decline in estrogen.[201]

Functions of DHEA/DHEAS

In adults, DHEA/DHEAS is thought to:

- Increase brain function
- Enhance the immune system
- Promote weight loss
- Stabilize mood
- Alleviate stress and anxiety
- Improve lipid profile

Changes in DHEA/DHEAS levels have been associated with changes in body composition with aging.[201]

DHEAS production is closely linked to levels of other hormones such as estradiol, progesterone, and testosterone.

Abnormal Adrenal Androgen Production

- **In menstruating women**: During the female menstrual cycle, there is a mid cycle dip in estradiol production just before ovulation. Within the same time frame there is a rise in testosterone level, increasing the libido. After ovulation, estrogen and progesterone rise again, "toning down" the testosterone effect. If there is not an appropriate progesterone and estrogen rise after day eighteen to twenty-eight, androgen effects inappropriately continue leading to symptoms of excess, such as acne and hirsutism among others.
- **During perimenopause and menopause**: Perimenopausal and menopausal women commonly develop acne and chin hair. This is thought to be from the adrenal glands making excess DHEA, which converts to testosterone, without the balancing effects from the ovarian progesterone and estradiol. How much testosterone comes from the adrenal glands versus the ovaries is debatable; however, similar symptoms also occur in women who have had their ovaries removed.

- **Postmenopause**: After menopause, many women become slightly more masculine; losing their feminine figure, developing coarser features, a balding hairline, and a slight change in voice. These women are usually otherwise healthy with strong, functional adrenal glands. The process is thought to be due to the adrenal glands "compensating" the ovarian decline. The ratio of estrogen, progesterone, and testosterone is changed after menopause. There is a higher ratio of DHEA and testosterone, lower estradiol and progesterone, and no ovarian rhythm.

Regulating DHEA/DHEAS

We do know that CRH and ACTH from the brain cause DHEA production to increase; however, we do not understand much more beyond this. We have no evidence of DHEA communicating back to the brain, although there is likely to be some mechanism; we have just not been able to identify it.

DHEA or Testosterone Replacement for Adrenal Dysfunction

To date, no trial or study has demonstrated the long-term safety of DHEA replacement,[202] or of testosterone replacement. It has been shown that oral DHEA administration in hypoadrenal women (women with low adrenal function) results in an unfavorable lipoprotein profile (cholesterol, triglycerides, and others).[203] However, more studies with topical administration and natural dosing need to be done.

Women with androgen deficiency due to pituitary dysfunction were studied after testosterone supplementation. Although they initially felt benefits such as psychological well-being, improved sexual function, improved bone mineral density and lean body mass, it was remarked that long-term safety data is lacking.[201]

Other studies have shown that, although the short-term improvements seen after androgen supplementation in newly diagnosed adrenal insufficiency patients leads to rapid and impressive improvement, well-being is often not fully restored and life expectancy may even be reduced.[202]

Many of the positive effects of DHEA such as bone mineral density improvements actually occur indirectly. DHEA converts to testosterone, which finally converts to estradiol, which has the above positive effects.[302]

Supplementing with DHEA without a rhythm may result in negative health consequences. Just as with any steroid, the initial feeling is good; only later do the negative consequences take effect.

It is difficult to get an accurate measure of DHEA production because DHEA does not last very long; therefore, most physicians get a DHEAS measurement instead.

It is important to understand that presently we do not clearly understand the long-term implications of adding DHEA or testosterone as an adrenal supplement.

Androstenedione

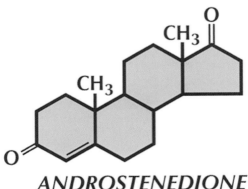

ANDROSTENEDIONE

Androstenedione is a hormone made in the adrenal glands and gonads of both male and females after about age eight. It is converted to other more potent hormones such as testosterone in tissues outside the adrenal gland. The androgenic effects of androstenedione and DHEA are mainly through their peripheral conversion to testosterone and DHT.[205]

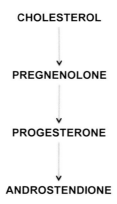

CHOLESTEROL

↓

PREGNENOLONE

↓

PROGESTERONE

↓

ANDROSTENDIONE

Illegal Use of Androstenedione

Androstenedione is also called "Andro" by athletes. It is a precursor to (in other words, it converts to) testosterone, which is used to build muscle and enhance performance. Andro, as well as other anabolic (muscle-building) steroids, have been prohibited by the International Olympic Committee and the National Collegiate Athletic Association for use in competition because of their life-threatening effects.[206]

Use of Anabolic (Body Building) Steroids

Taking anabolic steroids beyond the normal healthy range for a young individual causes long-term imbalance leading to dysfunction and poor health.

Even men in their twenties can develop liver dysfunction from the inappropriate use of testosterone and/or related steroids intended for body building.

Due to negative feedback, if external androgens are taken, the male gonads (testes) stop making testosterone, causing the testes to shrink. Eventually, sperm count drops, which affects future reproductive function. As mentioned earlier, this concept is used for male contraceptive development.

Cortisol

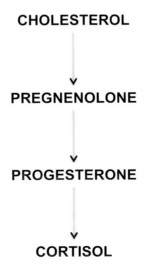

CH_2OH

$C = O$

OH

HO

O

CORTISOL

Cortisol is one of the most important hormones for life. It is made in the middle cortex of the adrenal glands. Cortisol, like all steroid hormones, is made from cholesterol. A healthy adrenal gland has the ability to make and store cholesterol ready to be converted into cortisol on demand.

The adrenal glands also have LDL and HDL receptors so that cholesterol (in the form of LDL and HDL) in the blood can enter and be stored to be used as needed.

CHOLESTEROL

↓

PREGNENOLONE

↓

PROGESTERONE

↓

CORTISOL

Cortisol Actions

Cortisol interacts closely with the neurotransmitters norepinephrine and epinephrine (adrenalin), which are made in the center of the adrenal gland for many critical functions; for example, to help in the inflammatory response.

Although it is generally known as the "stress" hormone, cortisol affects numerous organ systems and body functions. For example, cortisol:

- Regulates blood glucose (stimulates glucose production)
- Inhibits protein synthesis, increasing breakdown
- Helps with cardiac output
- Stimulates red blood cell production
- Suppresses the immune system
- Enhances the anti-inflammatory response
- Is involved in the bone marrow's response to injury or infection
- Decreases reproductive ability
- Decreases bone formation, inhibiting bone-forming actions
- Thins small blood vessel walls (enhances bruising)
- Impairs collagen formation, therefore thins skin
- Causes water retention (inhibits the water-eliminating hormone, ADH)
- In excess causes muscle weakness and pain
- Increases stomach acid production, increasing risk of ulcers
- Causes psychological disturbances when out of balance
- Causes insomnia when out of balance
- Is involved in energy production in the mitochondria

In the event of short-term stress, cortisol contributes to providing energy for the increased demands on the body. For example, glucose is quickly made available while the effects on the cardiovascular system ensure a timely cardiac response and the body is protected from unregulated inflammation.

Medical Uses of Cortisol (and its Derivatives)

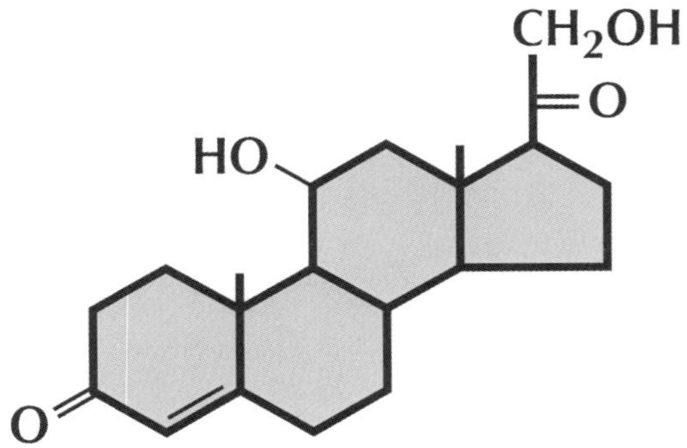

CH_2OH
=O
HO

O

CORTICOSTERONE

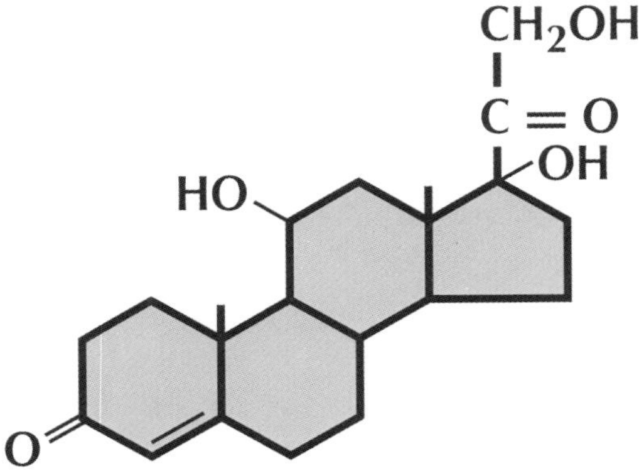

CH_2OH
C = O
OH
HO

O

CORTISOL

Cortisol has a relatively short life; it has many fates, including being reversibly converted to cortisone (Corticosterone). Cortisone is more stable and is used topically on the skin where it can be converted back to cortisol to reduce inflammation.

Many dermatologists still inject cortisol into acne pimples/cysts to reduce inflammation. Problems with this symptomatic approach include further damage to the skin, including a greater chance of scarring as well as thinning of the skin.

Many other preparations of cortisol-like products (corticosteroids) such as prednisone, methylprednisolone, and prednisolone are used medically because of their increased stability and ability to be converted to cortisol within the body.

Imbalances in Cortisol

Like all hormones, cortisol needs to be in balance. For example, too much or too little cortisol can have severe psychological symptoms. As with all steroids, there is an initial feeling of well-being, but prolonged excessive exposure can lead to emotional instability and depression.

Low cortisol levels can make a person feel irritable, apathetic, and depressed.[200] However, too much cortisol can also lead to many psychological disturbances, which are due to cortisol's direct action on the brain.[24]

Regulation of Cortisol Production

The brain operates on a set point or "thermostat" for cortisol levels. If the blood cortisol level is low, then CRH from the hypothalamus stimulates ACTH from the pituitary gland, which stimulates the adrenal glands to make more cortisol.[207]

Many other factors other than low cortisol influence CRH to produce more cortisol. Physical stress, mental stress, illnesses, and low blood sugar can all influence CRH. Too much cortisol, whether naturally created during chronic stress or given medically, induces obesity, insulin resistance, glucose intolerance, dyslipidemia (altered cholesterol profile), and high blood pressure.[208]

Natural Rhythm of Cortisol

CRH has a diurnal pattern of release, which results in cortisol levels rising during early morning, declining during the day, with a small rise in late afternoon. CRH and cortisol need to be released in the correct rhythm; otherwise the sleep/wake cycle becomes disturbed as well as many other functions in the body. The opposing hormone for cortisol is thought to be melatonin (See Chapter 27, Melatonin)

Cortisol Treatment

If cortisol is given by mouth or intravenously for an extended time, the adrenal glands stop making their own due to an interruption in the feedback loop. If cortisol treatment is discontinued, the adrenal glands recover after a few weeks.

"Safe Uses" of Cortisol

Many anti-aging physicians promote "safe uses" of cortisol by administering small doses to combat minor ailments such as colds and flu.

Other scientists discourage this practice because they believe that minor stress enhances survival by turning on "survival" genes. Either way, more studies are needed to clarify the best course of action.

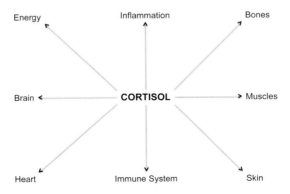

It is important to remember that too much or too little of any hormone or neurotransmitter can cause similar symptoms of imbalance.

Aldosterone

Aldosterone is a steroid hormone made in the outer cortex of the adrenal glands. Like all steroid hormones, aldosterone is made from cholesterol.

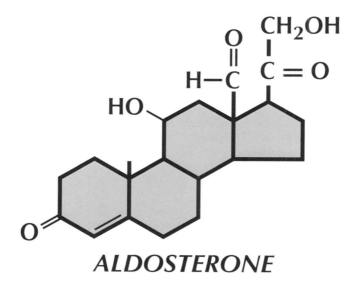

ALDOSTERONE

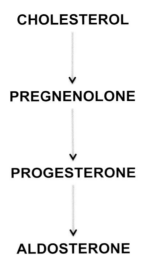

CHOLESTEROL

PREGNENOLONE

PROGESTERONE

ALDOSTERONE

The adrenal cortex zone, where aldosterone is made, has specific enzymes that make aldosterone from progesterone, rather than making the other adrenal steroids.

Functions of Aldosterone

Aldosterone is most recognized for regulating salt and water balance through its action on the kidneys. However, it also helps regulate salt and water balance in the colon, salivary glands, sweat glands, and the gastric glands.

ACTH regulates all adrenal steroids other than aldosterone. Aldosterone is mainly regulated by a substance called renin, which is released from the kidneys in response to blood pressure drop.

- A deficiency in aldosterone causes dehydration, salt wasting, and high levels of potassium.

- Too much aldosterone causes hypertension, decreased potassium, increased sodium, and water retention.

Diseases Associated with Aldosterone

There may be several reasons for very high levels of aldosterone. For example, aldosterone-secreting tumors can develop, which result in high salt and water retention, potassium depletion, high blood pressure, and weakness. It is therefore, important to identify the cause of recent onset high blood pressure. There are also several other congenital and acquired diseases of the adrenal glands that lead to inappropriate aldosterone secretion and disease.

Licorice and Cortisol

Cortisol has different effects on the body related to its concentration. High levels of cortisol mimic the effects of aldosterone on the kidneys, leading to high blood pressure and salt retention.

A substance in licorice (glycyrrhizic acid) has similar effects as too much cortisol or aldosterone on the kidneys, and can also cause high blood pressure.

Aldosterone and Aging

As the functions of the adrenal glands decline with age, aldosterone production also declines. This could result from the aging kidneys, the aging adrenal glands, or both.

Elderly individuals often complain of not retaining water after drinking it. If the problem is limited to the night, kidney dysfunction and diabetes is probably not the only cause; quite often the problem also lies in inadequate adrenal function.

The cortisol rise in early morning results in an urge to empty the bladder. During deep sleep, aldosterone should be reabsorbing water back from the kidneys so that the bladder does not fill too much too quickly and the body does not dehydrate. However, elderly individuals with dysfunctional adrenal glands usually have to urinate frequently during the night.

Treatment with Aldosterone

If the adrenal glands are not functioning well, aldosterone replacement should not be the first line of treatment. Aging individuals certainly need to optimize adrenal function, but this needs to be done very cautiously.

Clinical studies have shown that treatment with excess aldosterone in humans has a deleterious effect on the heart by being profibrotic; causing unfavorable remodeling of heart tissue, thereby increasing morbidity and mortality (dysfunction and death).[208]

Measuring Adrenal Function

Although there are no standard tests to measure the health and function of the adrenal glands, there are certain tests that can be helpful.

- When measuring any hormone, it is important to measure the hormone level at its peak.

- Cortisol is one of the most reliable tests of adrenal health and function. One of the main reasons is that we recognize that cortisol has a distinct daily rhythm; it is highest in early morning and lowest at late night.

- DHEAS is also a helpful indicator of adrenal health and function; it is measured rather than DHEA because of the short half-life of DHEA.

- There may be some monthly variation of DHEA and DHEAS production in menstruating women due to their menstrual cycle. However, this needs to be further understood.

Treatment

There is no medical consensus of how to treat diminished adrenal function. It is important to ensure a healthy diet with correct nutritional support and stress management before taking any further medical steps.

Adrenal steroids, like all steroid hormones, have a distinct dose response effect. The levels need to be balanced, as too much or too little will cause negative effects.[24]

Several academic centers around the world are involved in research on how to address adrenal dysfunction. At this point, the data is scattered and in preliminary stages; no concrete recommendations can be made.

Treatment with Pregnenolone

Some healthcare providers feel that small doses of pregnenolone help with the symptoms of adrenal fatigue, but not everyone can tolerate this. This is likely due to the different pathways pregnenolone takes.

When treating inadequate adrenal function, some important points to consider are:

- If the patient can tolerate pregnenolone, it can provide a significant relief of symptoms. The studies on pregnenolone supplementation are limited, but if one does take the supplement, the doses should be minimal, and should not be taken without a few days off per month, until further studies are available.

- In a depressed, agitated patient, small doses of pregnenolone can be a safer approach than antidepressants and sleep medications.

- In menstruating women, the adrenal glands seem to be the most active just prior to ovulation, as well as at the tail end of one cycle and the beginning of the next. However, there are no studies so far that have shown a clear rhythm.

- DHEA is not recommended for adrenal support before pregnenolone or progesterone has been tried. DHEA is one of the end products of the adrenal glands. Very little is known on how DHEA, DHEAS, or the hormones they convert to, may directly or indirectly feed back to the brain; therefore, supplementation may cause unpredictable consequences.

- Inadequate cholesterol in the body results in difficulty dealing with stress. Again, a healthy, balanced diet is necessary before considering any supplementation.

(See Chapter 23, Pregnenolone).

Adrenal Gland and Stress

One of the most indisputable facts in medicine is that stress is the number-one factor in predicting health.

The human stress-handling system is a complex interaction between the hormones and neurotransmitters of the brain and body.[24,209]

Stress affects men and women differently. Women of reproductive years who undergo sustained stress will see some change in their menstrual pattern, even if temporary. This is directly related to the adrenal-ovarian connection.

Men too suffer from inadequate adrenal gland function; however, their hormonal dynamics are different. In men, the main androgens come from the testes, so their dependence on the adrenal glands for androgens is less than in women, who rely very little on their ovaries for androgens.

Most types of stress, including physical and mental, affect CRH production and hence ACTH production, and therefore lead to increased cortisol and adrenal steroid production.

Short-term and long-term stress has many implications including:

- Reproduction issues and the outcome of pregnancy
- Skin problems such as acne

- Hair loss

- Fatigue

- Burden on brain neurotransmitters affecting sleep, memory, and mood as well as every other aspect of life.[206]

- There is no known function of health that is not adversely affected by stress.

What to avoid

Adrenal dysfunction can lead to feelings of stress and anxiety. This is not a justification for giving antidepressants or anxiolytic drugs. These drugs can certainly cause temporary relief and are FDA approved, but they are harmful in the long term. It is safer to understand where the natural imbalance is and correct that as safely as possible.

General Points about Adrenal Steroids

- All adrenal steroid hormones are made from cholesterol.

- If cholesterol is not available in the diet, the liver tries to make it from scratch. But still the liver can make only a certain amount.

- The cells need to be healthy to take in cholesterol and convert it to pregnenolone and the rest of the steroid hormones.

- High blood cholesterol is an indicator of suboptimal health because the cholesterol is not able to enter the cells and be utilized. True health is in utilization of cholesterol, not elimination.

- We do not understand the adrenal rhythm, other than the rhythmic stimulation from CRH and ACTH for cortisol production.

- Although every hormone is involved in the overall feedback system of the body, it is generally safer to treat with the one that is the highest in the chain, unless definitive information is available otherwise.

Future Studies

Other than cortisol, which depends on the brain for a daily rhythm, we do not clearly understand the rhythm for other adrenal hormones. We need to better understand how DHEA, DHEAS, androstenedione, testosterone, and DHT interact with the brain and gonads.

Of particular benefit would be to see well-designed studies on the polycystic ovary syndrome, which has serious health consequences for those affected, and is becoming increasingly prevalent.

Aldosterone supplementation needs further studying due to the reports of cardiac problems.

Chapter 23

Pregnenolone

Pregnenolone is made directly from cholesterol in the vital cell structures called mitochondria.

THE CELL (simplified)

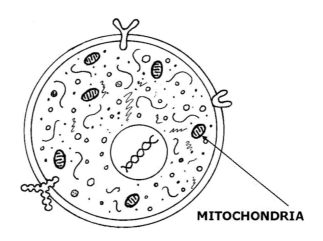

MITOCHONDRIA

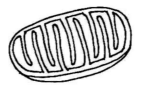

MITOCHONDRIA

In the pathway of steroid hormone synthesis, pregnenolone formation is the first and critical step.

Mitochondria deteriorate in number and function with aging, mainly from oxidative stress due to environmental damage and metabolic byproducts. This is one of the reasons that pregnenolone production decreases as we age.

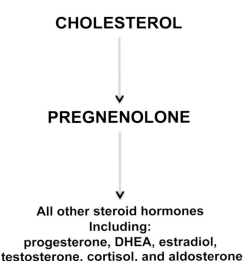

CHOLESTEROL

PREGNENOLONE

**All other steroid hormones
Including:
progesterone, DHEA, estradiol,
testosterone, cortisol, and aldosterone**

The adrenal glands, testes, and ovaries have typically been known to use cholesterol for making pregnenolone and the resulting hormones. Recently we have learned that the brain also has the capacity to use cholesterol for the synthesis of pregnenolone and its related hormones needed for critical functions in the brain.[28,31,29,30] We are learning that organs such as the heart can also make steroid hormones for local use.

Replacing Pregnenolone

The information on replacing pregnenolone is incomplete and under development. Considering that there are so many chemicals, hormones, and neurotransmitters, which all interact with each other for balancing the human system, it is imperative to replace hormones with utmost caution, with full regard to the available medical data.

See Adrenal Gland Treatment

Chapter 24

Thyroid Gland

A normal functioning thyroid gland is necessary for every aspect of normal growth, development, and heath.

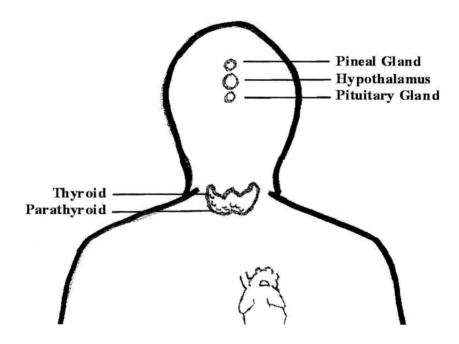

Pineal Gland
Hypothalamus
Pituitary Gland

Thyroid
Parathyroid

The thyroid gland is located in the front mid neck area (area of the "Adam's apple"). It has strong innervations (connections) from the nervous system as well as a very robust blood supply. The gland is very sensitive to viral infections, other hormone imbalances, and, importantly, high levels of stress.

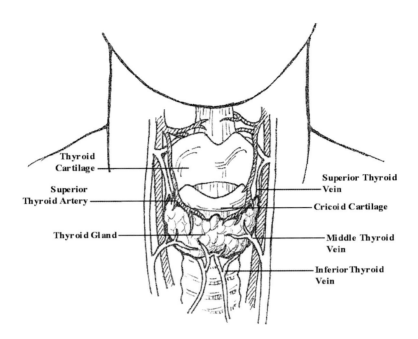

The thyroid gland is mainly recognized for producing thyroid hormone (T4). The gland also makes calcitonin, which has a role in inhibiting bone resorption.

Thyroid Hormone

Thyroid hormone is derived from an amino acid (tyrosine). Iodine is attached to the thyroid hormone within the gland. The number of iodine molecules and to which part of the thyroid hormone they are attached determines what type of thyroid hormone is produced. (i.e., T4, T3, T2, T1)

Many complex reactions take place within the thyroid gland, including the addition of iodine molecules to make and store the main thyroid hormone (T4).

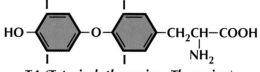

T4 (Tetraiodothyronine, Thyroxine)

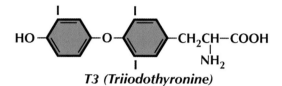

T3 (Triiodothyronine)

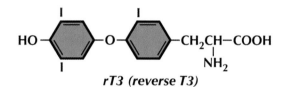

rT3 (reverse T3)

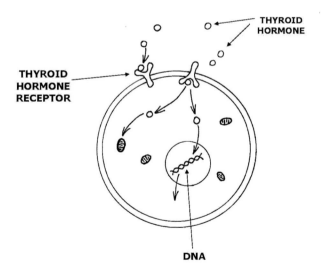

THYROID HORMONE ACTION ON THE CELL

- T4 is the inactive form of thyroid hormone. It is stored in several parts of the body and converted to the active form T3 as needed.

- The production of thyroid hormone T4 and its subsequent conversion to the active T3 is intricately controlled by countless factors including enzymes, chemical signals, iodine concentration, as well as adequate cell energy. We do not fully understand what triggers the conversion of the inactive T4 to the active T3.

- About 90 percent of the thyroid hormone exists as T4, and about 9 percent as T3. A small portion exists as an inactive form of T3 called reverse T3.

- The level of thyroid hormone varies during the day. T3 levels are typically greater in the morning. Although there is some variation in thyroid hormone production related to the ovarian cycle, less is known about the variation in men. Of note, though, is that men seem to have fewer thyroid deficiency complaints than women.

Age-related Changes in Thyroid Function

Thyroid hormone production diminishes as the thyroid gland ages.

As individuals deviate further away from their personal healthy range, symptoms follow, eventually leading to dysfunction and imbalance in other hormone systems.

Other than having a general rhythm, the thyroid gland also works on demand. We realize this due to the thyroid gland's intricate connection to the nervous system.

Often individuals, especially women, who have led physically or mentally stressful lives develop some level of thyroid dysfunction. Many suffer for years without treatment because they are still within the "normal" range in standard lab testing.

Standard-of-care medicine does not treat an under-functioning thyroid gland unless the lab values are outside the normal range. The "normal" range is an average for the population and is not adjusted for the individual.

Control of Thyroid Hormone

The brain (hypothalamus and pituitary) is closely involved in thyroid hormone balance; however, many other factors also contribute to a healthy functioning thyroid gland.

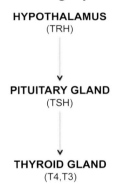

HYPOTHALAMUS
(TRH)

↓

PITUITARY GLAND
(TSH)

↓

THYROID GLAND
(T4,T3)

Storage and Release of Thyroid Hormone

Although thyroid hormone is made and stored in the thyroid gland, it is stored in other organs too. For example, about 30 percent of the body's T4 pool is stored in the liver and kidneys. These other storages sites act as additional sources of T4 to buffer the blood levels.

For this reason, taking thyroid supplement once a day is adequate because the conversion to T3 takes place as needed in an otherwise healthy system.

Functions of Thyroid Hormone

At different developmental stages, thyroid hormone serves different functions. The fetus needs adequate thyroid hormone for development and depends on the mother to be thyroid balanced.

Throughout life, the thyroid hormone affects well-being and is necessary for every aspect of growth and development.

We should be aware that thyroid function is intricately connected to every other function and hormone system in the body. An imbalance in the thyroid system ultimately affects other critical functions in the body.

Some of the actions of thyroid hormone

- Cell function, basic metabolic rate, and metabolism require thyroid hormone balance.

- Studies have shown that thyroid hormone receptors exist on the mitochondria demonstrating the critical role of thyroid hormone in energy production.[83,84,85,86]

- The functioning, maturation, and balance of every organ system including the liver, heart, and kidneys is dependent on thyroid balance.[211,212,213,214,215,216]

- Thyroid hormone stimulates fat synthesis and breakdown.

- Thyroid hormone affects protein synthesis and breakdown (i.e., protein turnover).

- Thyroid hormone affects the body's lipid balance (metabolism), affecting levels of triglycerides, cholesterol, and LDL receptors among others.[217]

- Thyroid hormone is needed for absorption and utilization of glucose, and therefore affects insulin activity.

- Thyroid hormone has a direct action on muscle movement.

- Thyroid hormone is critical for normal brain and nervous system development, maturation, and function, including neurogeneration, cognition, and mood balance.[218,219,220,221,222]

- Thyroid hormone closely interacts with other hormones including insulin and steroid hormones.[127]

- Thyroid hormone is important for healthy scalp hair including hair pigmentation.[101]

- Thyroid hormone has an important role in balancing skin function including moisture and pigmentation. Melasma, which is a genetic condition of patchy areas of hyperpigmentation, worsens with low thyroid function.[293]

Hypothyroidism (Low Thyroid Function)

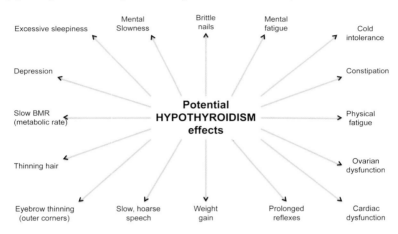

The effects of hypothyroidism do not occur overnight or all at once. Because hormones work in synchrony with one another, it is likely that a hormone inadequacy in one gland has an effect on the production and functioning of another.

Causes of Hypothyroidism

Other than age-related decline in thyroid function, hypothyroidism can be caused by factors such as:

- Autoimmune conditions, including Hashimoto's thyroiditis
- Other thyroid inflammatory conditions
- Cancer
- Radiation exposure

- Iodine deficiency
- Medications
- Defects in the hormone-producing pathway
- Inadequate production of other hormones
- Too much iodine, which causes a block in effective thyroid hormone synthesis (Wolff-Chaikoff effect)

Measuring Low Thyroid Function

While measuring blood levels for suspicion of hypothyroidism, it is not sufficient to measure TSH and T4.

The minimum blood tests should be:

- TSH
- FreeT4
- FreeT3

It is important to understand that every person has his or her individual optimum level of thyroid hormone. What is normal for one person may be too high or too low for the other.

A person will become progressively more symptomatic as his or her thyroid function deviates away from his or her personal normal range.

Antibodies

Many patients have had undocumented incidences of thyroid conditions which invalidate the measurement of TSH. In such cases, further testing, for example, for thyroid antibodies is needed.

Reverse T3 (rT3)

Other less-common problems include normal TSH, T4, normal antibodies, but, for some reason, incorrect conversion of T4 to free T3. There may be plenty of T3, but, with the wrong iodine molecule being removed, rT3 (reverse T3) is made instead of Free T3. The patient is symptomatic, but the lab results are "normal."

Hyperthyroidism (Overactive Thyroid Function)

Excess thyroid hormone is usually due to diseases such as Graves disease where there is over stimulation of the thyroid gland.

Because thyroid hormone has similar effects as the sympathetic nervous system, too much thyroid hormone causes symptoms such as increase in heart rate, excess sweating, and tremor.

Graves' disease

Graves' disease is a disease of the immune system (an autoimmune disorder), with some genetic predisposition.

Typical symptoms are a goiter (enlarged thyroid gland), as well other symptoms including those of hyperthyroidism listed below.

Many times, a person treated for Graves' disease will be become hypothyroid, a condition much easier to treat.

Some symptoms of Hyperthyroidism

- Increased heat production with heat intolerance
- Cardiac changes including fast heart rate and palpitations
- Tiredness, fatigue
- Tremor and nervousness
- Skin changes
- Eye problems, including enlarged bulging eyes
- Increase in appetite

Other Significant Thyroid Conditions

Wolff-Chaikoff Effect

In the Wolff-Chaikoff Effect, too much iodine in a normal thyroid gland inhibits adequate thyroid hormone synthesis. This is one reason it is important not to overuse iodine supplements.

Thyroiditis

Thyroiditis (inflammation of the thyroid gland) can result after a viral infection. Initially, the symptoms are those of hyperthyroidism, followed by transient hypothyroidism. Although this usually resolves on its own, it can also result in permanent hypothyroidism.

Treating Underactive Thyroid (Hypothyroidism)

There are several cautions to treating low thyroid; for example:

- If there is suspicion of adrenal insufficiency, giving thyroid supplements can be dangerous without first correcting the adrenal insufficiency.

- Individuals with cardiac dysfunction should be monitored very carefully.

Although the thyroid gland, like anything else, decreases in function with ageing, it is useful to have a medical evaluation to rule out other metabolic deficiencies including gonadal (ovary and testes) dysfunctions.

Standard of Care Treatment for Hypothyroidism

The administration of levothyroxine sodium (T4) is the standard medical treatment for low thyroid function. This is sold under the trade name Synthroid®. Several generic versions of levothyroxine sodium are available, for example, Levothyroxine, Levoxyl, and Levothyroid. There is very little difference between these versions; and no significant data to support the use of one form over the other.

The medical choice of treating low thyroid with levothyroxine sodium is reasonable for now. However, the threshold for treatment initiation is outdated, inadequate, and needs to be revised. More accurate lab reference levels are needed, and the symptoms of the patient must be considered.

It is usually recommended that levothyroxine sodium products be taken it in the morning on an empty stomach. The stomach is best empty for maximum absorption. However, it depends on the individual as to whether morning or night is better. Not enough research has been done on this topic. In reality, it may not even matter. The rationale for morning dosing is that thyroid activity is greatest in the morning. However, the body does not always immediately convert T4 to T3 once it is ingested. Furthermore, we do not know exactly what signals the conversion.

Armour Thyroid

Armour Thyroid is derived and prepared from pig tissue. It is called "natural" because it occurs in nature. Armour thyroid consists of T4, T3, T2 and T1, whereas levothyroxine consists of only T4. A few points about Armour thyroid:

- The medical community is less comfortable with dosing Armour thyroid because it was never included in the standard-of-care protocol. It is difficult to find a medical or endocrinology text that adequately describes the uses of Armour thyroid.

- Many patients believe Armour thyroid is better because it is "natural." Armour thyroid's source is natural; it is then further modified in a lab. However, what is natural to a pig is not natural to a human.

- A patient may initially feel better on Armour thyroid than he or she did on T4 (any form of levothyroxine sodium). This phenomenon is more often than not temporary and usually occurs if the patient was inadequately treated with T4, or if the patient is unable to convert T4 to T3, the active form of the hormone.

- A healthy body knows when to convert T4 to T3. This conversion is not a random process, and we understand very little of what signals control this tightly regulated system. It is not medically sound to administer a potent active hormone such as T3 when so little is known about its conversion from T4.

- Armour thyroid has T2 and T1 in ratios natural to pigs; we do not know what the long-term implications of T1 and T2 supplementation are.

Before supplementing with Armour thyroid it would be an option to first:

- Optimize T4 supplementation
- Take a few days off a month (until we know more about the thyroid rhythm, as no hormone is made in a constant dose)
- Optimize the levels of all other hormone systems

Cytomel

Cytomel is T3. Some doctors give this in very small doses when patients complain of being symptomatic on T4 alone. As mentioned earlier, T3 is the active, potent form of T4, and we do not know what signals T4-to-T3 conversion. We do know that T3 and T4 levels fluctuate during the day.

It is advisable to make sure that the body's stores of T4 are adequate, and other hormones are evaluated before T3 replacement is considered.

If the body does not produce adequate T3, there could be many medical reasons, which need to be evaluated. Treating the underlying cause is better than taking potent pharmaceuticals with little scientific basis and unknown consequences.

Points to Keep in Mind when Replacing Thyroid Hormone

- All hormones, including thyroid hormone, have a rhythm and communicate intricately with other hormones and neurotransmitters in the body.

- Initially, almost all hormones give a feeling of well-being when replaced; however, if the replacement is unnatural to the body, eventually the body system becomes confused and inefficient.

- Although, as mentioned above, it is reasonable to take T4 at night, as it takes time to convert to T3, Armour thyroid should only be taken in the morning as it has T3, which makes it difficult to sleep due to stimulatory effects.

Treating Overactive Thyroid (Hyperthyroidism)

Hyperthyroidism is, at least in the short term, a more medically serious and complicated condition than hypothyroidism. Hyperthyroidism is not typically a disease of aging; therefore, it is managed by standard medicine protocol by endocrinologists.

General Points about Thyroid Management

- Often when patients experience symptoms of low energy, depression, weight gain, poor sleep, irritability, hair loss, and feeling cold, blood tests come back "normal," and the diagnosis of thyroid dysfunction is dismissed. It is common that, if the patient is persistent, he or she will be offered antidepressants, and told to eat less and exercise more.

- The diagnosis should be pursued with further thyroid testing as well as checking other hormone systems.

- Healthy thyroid function is critical for health. Humans are designed to have symptoms when something is not balanced. Neglecting to optimize a low thyroid function will lead to further deterioration in health.

- Physicians often fear that over treating thyroid will lead to bone loss and heart arrhythmias (irregular heart beat). This is based on the observation that hyperthyroidism causes these symptoms. However, it takes a lot of T4 (not Armour or T3) to overdose on thyroid hormone.

- Low thyroid has been shown to have detrimental effects on cardiac function. Bone loss, which occurs more commonly with estrogen deficiency due to ovarian decline, can be monitored with routine dual energy X-ray absorptiometry (DEXA) scans.

- If suboptimal hormone levels are suspected but blood tests return "normal," the tests should be repeated at a different time within the next few months before dismissing the problem.

- Thyroid hormones including T4 and T3 have some rhythm. In women, thyroid hormone levels seem to be synchronized with the ovarian cycle. The synchrony with male hormones is less well understood. More data is needed before specific recommendations can be made. However, because no hormone is made in a continuous dose, it may be helpful to take a few days off in the month.

Chapter 25

Growth Hormone

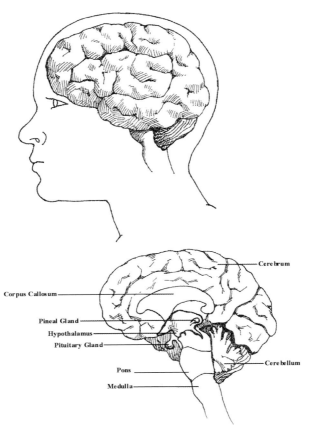

Growth hormone is also referred to as HGH (human growth hormone). It is a protein hormone made in the section of the brain called the pituitary gland. The release of HGH from the brain occurs in a pulsatile manner. Growth hormone is necessary for correct growth, development, and maintenance of health.

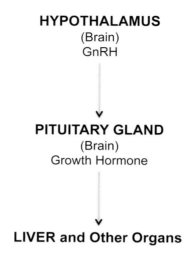

HYPOTHALAMUS
(Brain)
GnRH

PITUITARY GLAND
(Brain)
Growth Hormone

LIVER and Other Organs

HGH in Children

In children, growth hormone is necessary for the proper growth and development of the body. Children with insufficient growth hormone, or who have growth hormone resistance, experience stunted growth or dwarfism.[223]

Too much growth hormone in children during their growth phase results in gigantism (acgromegaly). Children with this disorder are usually of normal weight and size at birth but experience abnormal growth thereafter. In the past, this condition went untreated to a point that a height in excess of eight feet could be reached.

HGH in Adults

In adults, a balance of growth hormone is necessary for the proper functioning of the body.[223]

Excessive growth hormone in adults results in an increase in the size of certain bones (flat bones), such as the skull, hands, feet, and face without increase in height.

Some of the effects of too much growth hormone result in dysfunctions that are similar to those that result from having too little.[225] Part of the reason could be that, unless a hormone is released in the correct dose and rhythm, the effects are diminished.

Too much or too little growth hormone in adults results in a lower quality of life, including altered body composition with reduced muscle mass, excess fat, reduced ability to walk quickly for prolonged length of time, and excessive fatigue among other symptoms.[225]

Functions of Normal Levels of Growth Hormone

Body Composition, Insulin Resistance, and Lipid Profile

Individuals with low levels of growth hormone were shown to have an overall improvement in metabolic functions after growth hormone treatment. Growth hormone has also been shown to increase lean body mass, increase fat loss, and improve lipid profile and insulin resistance in obese individuals with functional growth hormone deficiency.[226,301]

Studies have shown that testosterone's effect on improving body composition in older men is enhanced by growth hormone supplementation.[227,228,229,230]

However, studies also show that, although growth hormone increases lean body mass, the functional capacity of the muscle is enhanced with the addition of physical training.[225, 231]

Brain

Growth hormone has many effects on the balance of brain function. Certain drug-resistant seizure disorders have shown improvement with growth hormone treatment.[232]

Memory, mood, psychological well-being, self-esteem, and mental fatigue have all been shown to improve with growth hormone replacement in adults with growth hormone deficiency.[233, 234]

Studies have shown that adults with severe growth hormone deficiency have impaired psychological and physical well-being, which benefits with growth hormone therapy.[235]

Cell Cycle

Correct cell division and function is essential for balanced functioning of the body. Growth hormone plays an important role in regulating cell division.[236]

Cell Health

Growth hormone and insulin-like growth factor 1 (IGF-1) are involved in balancing free radicals and curtailing oxidative stress.[237]

Oxidative stress is a term that reflects a damaging environment in the cell. Chemical reactions are constantly taking place in the cells, producing highly charged, bullet-like molecules called free radicals as byproducts. A small amount of free radicals are necessary to "ignite" further cell reactions. Damage by free radicals is usually taken care of by the cell's inbuilt damage repair system. But, over time, there is more damage than repair, which is referred to as oxidative stress.

Chronic Pain

In clinical trials, patients with chronic pain, fibromyalgia, and fatigue have been shown to benefit from growth hormone therapy.[238]

Tissue Regeneration and Maintenance

Growth hormone has an important role in the regeneration of tissue growth and maintenance; for example, survival of special retinal nerve cells in the eye is regulated via growth hormone.[238]

The thymus gland, which has immune-related functions in adults, relies on the GH-to-IGF axis for normal maintenance.[240]

Factors Affecting Growth Hormone Release

Growth hormone function is dependent on its pulsatile secretion, which is regulated in a complex manner. Many factors affect the pulsatile secretion of growth hormone, including estradiol, testosterone, body fat (percentage), and age.[88,241,242,243,244] There are also other proteins and hormones that affect the release of growth hormone.[223]

Growth hormone is a protein hormone and is therefore dependent on cell receptors to enter the cells; estrogen increases receptors for growth hormone. Administering growth hormone without first replacing estrogen in women and testosterone in men does not give an optimum result.

Measuring Growth Hormone

Growth hormone has a very short half-life; it gets broken down quickly. Also, the pulsatile nature of its release makes getting an accurate measurement challenging. However, growth hormone directly stimulates release of IGF-1 from the liver, which exists in a more constant level in the blood; therefore, IGF-1 levels are used as an indicator of growth hormone status.[245, 246]

Growth Hormone Replacement

Legal Issues

Growth hormone misuse and abuse by athletes caused its use to be more tightly regulated than any other hormone. This followed the publication of an important study showing the benefits of growth hormone replacement in men over sixty.[226]

The government has banned the use of growth hormone for any use other than a documented deficiency in the production and release of growth hormone from the brain (pituitary gland).

Unfortunately, the measurements required for evaluating the

pituitary release of growth hormone and the criteria for deficiency are insufficient, outdated, and do not keep in consideration age related decline.

Illegal Uses

HGH is the only bioidentical hormone that cannot be used "off label" (which means, it cannot be used for any purpose other than what is allowed by the FDA).This has led to its illegal use; it can be acquired illegally from the internet. Also, many physicians have lost their licenses because of "off label" prescription of HGH.

Several variations of HGH are available over the internet. Due to the potential benefits, substandard products have been also produced. Also, due to the legal implications, consumers use HGH without checking blood levels, putting their health at risk.

Cautions

Growth hormone functions appropriately only if it is released or administered in a pulsatile manner.[246]

Growth hormone replacement should not be undertaken before the adrenal and thyroid glands are evaluated to avoid worsening symptoms of incipient (developing) adrenal insufficiency and hypothyroidism.[154]

Approved Uses

IGF-1 is approved by the FDA for children who have growth deficiencies and who meet treatment criteria.[248]

Growth hormone can be replaced subcutaneously (by injection) or inhalation. Studies in children have shown that delivery of growth hormone via deep lung through inhalation to be feasible.[249]

Individuals should undergo specific testing to demonstrate a defect in the production and release of growth hormone from the brain before growth hormone is administered.

Chapter 26

Vitamin D

Over the past few years, there has been a heightened awareness of the numerous crucial functions of vitamin D. The scientific literature on the benefits of adequate vitamin D is extensive and continues to grow.

Terminology

Although vitamin D has always been considered a vitamin, there are still conflicting arguments as to its true definition. Some sources insist that it is indeed a vitamin,[250] while others call it a hormone or prohormone (a precursor to a hormone).

- Vitamin D broadly refers to a group of related compounds.

- The biologically active form of vitamin D is chemically known as 1,25-dihydoxycholecalciferol, also referred to as calcitriol or simply Vitamin D3.

- Vitamin D3 can be activated only through the liver and kidneys.

Vitamin D may not fit well into any definition, but its benefits are crucial for health and need to be understood.

Sources of Vitamin D

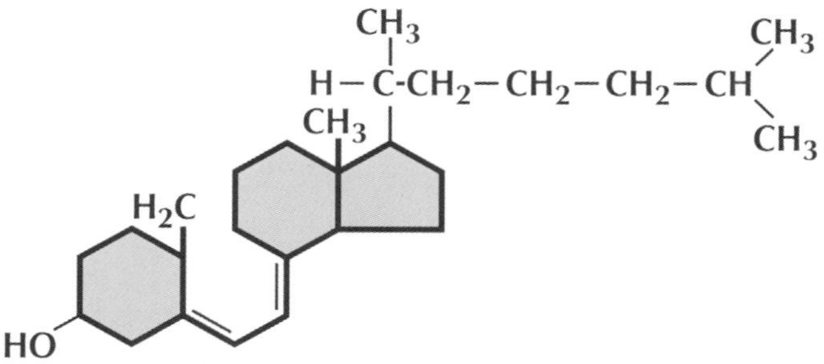

$$\text{HO} - \text{...} \quad \underset{|}{H - \overset{CH_3}{\underset{CH_3}{C}} - CH_2 - CH_2 - CH_2 - CH} \overset{CH_3}{\underset{CH_3}{\diagdown}}$$

H₂C

D3 (VITAMIN D3, CHOLECALCIFEROL)

Vitamin D is either made completely in the body or obtained from the diet. As mentioned above, Vitamin D from either diet or body has to be activated through the liver and kidneys for the final biologically active product.

Diet

- Dietary vitamin D comes from plant or animal sources.

- Animal sources eventually become activated once modified through the liver and kidneys. Typical animal sources are fish, fish oil, eggs, and beef. Dairy products containing cholesterol can also become a source for vitamin D.

- Certain plants, fungi, and mushrooms contain vitamin D2, but this is not a significant source.

Body

- In the body, a cholesterol-like molecule (7-dehydrocholesterol) is activated by sunlight through the skin. This is then further activated through the liver and kidneys for the final activated form.

Benefits of Vitamin D3

Bone

One of the most recognized functions of vitamin D3 is its role in calcium balance in the blood and absorption of calcium from the gut.

The active form of vitamin D3 is involved in regulating bone metabolism, calcium, and phosphate balance, as well as balancing cell and tissue growth. [251,252]

Studies have shown that vegetarian children do not have adequate levels of vitamin D in the blood in winter months, which could lead to disturbances in bone metabolism.[253]

A study showed a greater incidence of metabolic bone disease in breast cancer survivors with low vitamin D levels.[254]

Insulin Resistance Diabetes

Vitamin D plays an important role in the utilization of glucose and the balance of metabolism. A recent study showed a link between low vitamin D levels, the metabolic syndrome, and insulin resistance in middle-aged and elderly individuals.[255,256]

Cardiovascular System

Vitamin D is shown to have substantial benefits in coronary heart disease, cardiovascular health, and cholesterol balance.[251,255,257,258,259] Blood pressure has been inversely related to vitamin D levels.[258]

Cancer

Many studies have shown the relationship between low vitamin D and cancer:

- There is increasing data to demonstrate the beneficial effects of vitamin D on cancer prevention.[259]

- Low vitamin D levels have been linked to many cancers including colorectal, pancreatic, endometrial, lung, ovarian, and breast cancer as well as multiple myeloma.[251,255,261,262,263]

- Recently, several studies have linked high levels of vitamin D3 to lower breast cancer risks,[263,264] and suggest that a deficiency in vitamin D is associated with poor survival.[265]

- Malignant melanoma has been shown to be more aggressive in vitamin D deficient patients.[266]

- Higher mortality has been documented in patients with colorectal cancer who have low vitamin D levels.[267]

- Studies have shown that vitamin D can slow down the rate of prostate-specific antigen (PSA) rise in patients with prostate cancer. This has lead researchers to investigate the role of vitamin D–related treatment for the prevention of prostate cancer.[268,269]

- Vitamin D was shown to increase apoptosis (death) of tumor cells in laryngeal carcinoma.[270]

Skin

Vitamin D has been linked to normal functioning of the skin. Different forms of vitamin D have been evaluated for the treatment of psoriasis.[251]

Musculoskeletal System

Studies have shown Vitamin D to be beneficial in musculoskeletal health by reducing pain and disability.[271] In some cases, low vitamin D levels have caused symptoms leading to the misdiagnosis of fibromyalgia.

A study from Saudi Arabia showed remarkable recovery after vitamin D deficiency–related muscle weakness was treated with vitamin D and calcium.[272]

Immune System

Vitamin D has a crucial role in balancing the immune system. The mechanism is thought to be by helping the body fight microbes while preventing excess inflammation.[257,273]

Studies have shown that vitamin D is necessary to fight seasonal viruses, and that it reduces respiratory infections in children.[274] Many anti-aging physicians advocate vitamin D supplements for the prevention of and curtailing of viral infections.

Mood

Vitamin D has been linked to mood stabilization; a deficiency is associated with seasonal affective disorder.[275,276]

Studies have also shown a link between cognitive impairment and vitamin D deficiency.[297]

Folic Acid

Folic acid is critical for countless areas of cell function including DNA and protein synthesis, cell division, and neurological function. Vitamin D has been shown to enhance gut absorption and cell uptake of folic acid.[277]

Measuring Vitamin D

There are many different forms of vitamin D. The active form of vitamin D is short lived. However, the partially activated form, 25-hydroxycholecalciferol, is the most prevalent in the body, and has the longest life before it is finally activated through the kidneys.

Dosing and Treatment

Vitamin D supplements should be in the form of vitamin D3. This will become activated once it is modified through the liver and kidneys.

The world consensus on how much vitamin D to use as a supplement is not clear and changes often. The daily dose typically recommended is 1000 IU to maintain a healthy level of vitamin D in the blood.[255] Doses between 1000 IU and 4000 IU per day have been recommended for cancer prevention.[262]

Recently, the baseline recommended doses have been increased for prevention of flu in the flu season.

Vitamin D is lipid soluble; therefore, oil based capsules may provide better absorption.

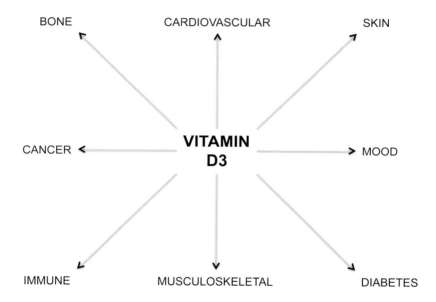

BONE   CARDIOVASCULAR   SKIN

CANCER   **VITAMIN D3**   MOOD

IMMUNE   MUSCULOSKELETAL   DIABETES

Chapter 27

Melatonin

Melatonin is produced in the brain in a tiny gland called the pineal gland.

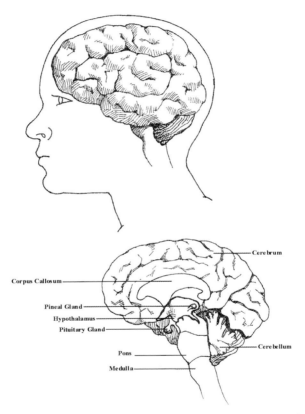

Melatonin is released at night and is secreted while we sleep. This release, coinciding with the body's circadian rhythm (rhythm related to a twenty-four-hour cycle) is critical to the optimum benefits of melatonin, and the other hormones it interacts with.

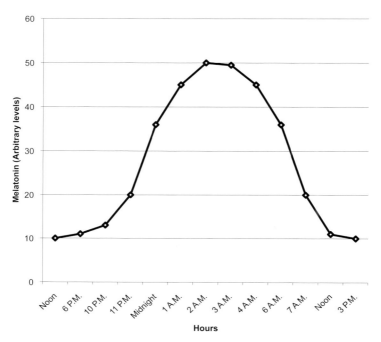

The pineal gland and melatonin

Functions of Melatonin

- Melatonin is recognized mostly as the hormone that sets the brain's biological clock, acting as a chemical messenger transmitting information about light-dark cycles. [278]

- For years, melatonin has been widely available over the counter as a sleep aid and for the treatment of jet lag.

- Changes in the circadian rhythm of natural melatonin have been linked to depression and other psychiatric illnesses, impairment of daily functioning, and cognitive decline.[279,280]

- Studies have shown the promising benefits of melatonin for use in individuals with severe circadian sleep disturbances and chronic sleep disorders.[281]

- Melatonin is shown to be a powerful antioxidant, and anti-inflammatory.[278,282]

- Studies have shown that the anti-inflammatory and antioxidative effects of melatonin are involved in the protection against vascular disease.[282]

- Melatonin has been shown to have important antioxidant effects in protecting nerve cells in the brain and retinal pigment cells in the eye.[283,284]

- Studies have linked impaired melatonin production and lack of its rhythm with several diseases including disorders of the digestive tract, the cardiovascular system, and insomnia.[285]

- Many studies are ongoing to understand the cancer protective and other benefits of melatonin.

- A recent study showed injection of melatonin locally decreased the severity of acute pancreatitis.[286]

Treatment

Like any other hormone, melatonin levels beyond physiological ranges can have negative effects, and, like any hormone, replacement, should be undertaken cautiously.

More studies are needed to understand correct dosing of melatonin.

Bibliography

1.   Tu K, Chen Z, Lipscombe L.L. Prevalence and incidence
        of hypertension from 1995 to 2005: a population-based
        study. *CMAJ.* 2008; 178(11):1429-1435.

2.   Kirtland KA, Geiss LS, Thompson TJ. State-Specific
        Incidence of Diabetes among Adults-Participating States,
        1995-1997 and 2005-2007. *JAMA.* 2008; 300(24):2847-
        2849.

3.   Olfson M, Marcus SC. National patterns in antidepressant
        medication treatment. *Arch Gen Psychiatry.* 2009;
        66(8):848-56.

4.   Kuo Y-F, Sharma G, Freeman JL, Goodwin JS. Growth
        in the care of older patients by hospitalists in the United
        States. *N Engl J Med.* 2009; 360:1102.

5.   Hamel MB, Drazen JM, Epstein AM. The growth of
        hospitalists and the changing face of primary care. *N
        Engl J Med.* 2009; 360:1141.

6.   Lobo RA. Clinical Review27 Effects of Hormone
        Replacement on Lipids and Lipoproteins in
        Postmenopausal Women. *J Clin Endocr Metab.* 1991;
        73(5):925-930.

7.   Zerr-Fouineau M, Jourdain M, Boesch C, Hecker M,
        Bronner C, Schini-Kerth VB. Certain Progestins Prevent
        the Enhancing Effect on 17ß-Estradiol on NO-Mediated
        Inhibition of Platelet Aggregation by Endothelial Cells.
        Arteriosclerosis, Thrombosis, and Vascular Biology.
        2009; 29:586-593.

8.   Stavrena DA, Wiench M, John S, Conway-Campbell
        BL, et al. Ultradian hormone stimulation induces
        glucocorticoid receptor-mediated pulses of gene

transcription. *Nat Cell Biol.* 2009; 11:1093-1102.

9.   Stefanidou M, Maravelius C, Spiliopoulou C. Human Exposure to Endocrine Disruptors and Breast Milk. *Endocr Metab Immune Disord Drug Targets.* 2009; 9(3):269-276

10. Ghisari M, Bonefeld-Jorgensen EC. Effects of plasticizers and their mixtures on estrogen receptor and thyroid hormone functions. *Toxic Lett.* 2009; 189(1):67-77.

11. Uzma N, Salar BM, Kumar BS, Aziz N, David MA, Reddy VD. Impact of organic solvents and environmental pollutants on the physiological function in petrol filling workers. *Int J Environ Res Public Health.* 2008; 5(3):139-46.

12. Doumouchtsis KK, Doumouchtsis SK, Doumouchtsis EK, Perrea DN. The effect of lead intoxication on endocrine functions. *Endocrinol Invest.* 2009; 32(2):175-83.

13. Heimier RA, Das B, Buchholz DR, Shi YB. The xenoestrogens bisphenol A inhibits postembryonic vertebrate development by antagonizing gene regulation by thyroid hormone. *Endocrinology.* 2009; 150(6):2964-73.

14. Fukai S, Akishita M. Hormone replacement therapy - growth hormone, melatonin, DHEA and sex hormones. *Nippon Rinsho.* 2009; 67(7):1396-401.

15. Strauss JF 3rd, Kallen CB, Christenson LK, et al. The steroidogenic acute regulatory protein (StAR): a window into the complexities of intracellular cholesterol trafficking. *Recent Prog Horm Res.* 1999; 54:369-94.

16. Demonacos CV, Karayanni N, Hatzoglou E, Tsiriyiotis C, Spandidos DA, Sekeris CE. Mitochondrial genes as

sites of primary action of steroid hormones. *Steroids*. 1996; 61(4):226-32.

17. Gutierrez J, Ballinger SW, Darley-Usmar VM, Lander A. Free radicals, mitochondria, and oxidized lipids: the emerging role in signal transduction in vascular cells. *Circ. Res*. 2006; 99(9):924-32.

18. Wallace KB, Starkov AA. Mitochondrial Targets of Drug Toxicity. *Annual Review of Pharmacology and Toxicology*. 2000; 40:353-388.

19. Bose M, Whittal RM, Gairola CG, Bose HS. *Toxicol Appl Pharmacol*. 2008; 229(1):56-64.

20. Roepke TA, Xue C, Bosch MA, Scalan TS, Kelly MJ, Rønnekleiv OK. Genes Associated with Membrane-Initiated Signaling of Estrogen and Energy Homeostasis. *Endocrinology*. 2008; 149(12):6113-6124.

21. Hammes SR, Levin ER. Extranuclear Steroid Receptors: Nature and Actions. *Endocr Rev*. 2007; 28(7):726-741

22. Vasudevan N, Pfaff DW. Membrane-Initiated Actions of Estrogens in Neuroendocrinology: Emerging Principles. *Endocr Rev*. 2007; 28(1):1-19.

23. Tasker JG, Di S, Malcher-Lopes R. Rapid Glucocorticoid Signaling via Membrane-Associated Receptors. *Endocrinology*. 2006; 147(12):5549-5556.

24. Prager EM, Johnson LR. Stress at the Synapse: Signal Transduction Mechanisms of Adrenal Steroids at Neuronal Membranes. *Sci Signal*. 2009; 2(86)

25. Edward DP. Regulation of signal transduction pathways by estrogen and progesterone. *Annu Rev Physiol*. 2005; 67:335-76.

26. Boonyaratanakornkit V, Edwards DP. Receptor mechanisms mediating non-genomic actions of sex

steroids. *Semin Reprod Med.* 2007; 25(3):139-53.

27. Simoncini T, Mannella P, Fornari L, Caruso A, Varone G, Genazzani AR. Genomic and non-genomic effects of estrogens on endothelial cells. *Steroids.* 2004; 69(8-9):537-42.

28. Whittaker MT, Gibbs TT, Farb DH. Pregnenolone sulfate induces NMDA receptor dependant release of dopamine from synaptic terminals in the striatum. *J Neurochem.* 2008; 107(2):510-21.

29. Sadri-Vakili G, Janis GC, Pierce RC, Gibbs TT, Farb DH. Nanomolar concentrations of pregnenolone sulfate enhances striatal dopamine overflow in vivo. *J Pharmacol Exp Ther.* 2008; 327(3):840-5.

30. Tsutsui K. Neurosteroids in the Purkinje cell: biosynthesis, mode of action and functional significance. *Mol Neurobiol.* 2008; 37(2-3):116-25.

31. Mellon SH. Neurosteroid regulation of central nervous system development. *Pharmacol Ther.* 2007; 116(1):107-24.

32. Porterfield SP, White BA. *Endocrine Physiology.* 3rd ed. Mosby, Inc; 2007: 223.

33. 33. Porterfield SP, White BA. *Endocrine Physiology.* 3rd ed. Mosby, Inc; 2007: 227

34. Chu MC, Rath KM, Huie J, Taylor HS. Elevated basal FSH in normal cycling women is associated with unfavorable lipid levels and increased cardiovascular risk. *Hum Reprod.* 2003; 18(8):1570-1573.

35. Gardner DG, Shoback D. *Greenspan's Basic & Clinical Endocrinology.* 8th ed. McGraw-Hill Companies, Inc; 2007: 506

36. Creus M, Peñarrubia J, Fábregues F, Vidal E, Carmona

F, Casamitjana R, Vanrell JA, Balasch J. Day 3 serum inhibin B and FSH and age as predictors of assisted reproduction treatment outcome. *Hum Reprod.* 2000; 15(11):2341-2346.

37. Gardner DG, Shoback D. *Greenspan's Basic & Clinical Endocrinology.* 8th ed. McGraw-Hill Companies, Inc; 2007: 515.

38. Porterfield SP, White BA. *Endocrine Physiology.* 3rd ed. Mosby, Inc; 2007: 234

39. Sztmanski LM, Bacon JL. Estrogen Therapy. emedicine from WebMD. Updated:Oct 20, 2008

40. Gardner DG, Shoback D. *Greenspan's Basic & Clinical Endocrinology.* 8th ed. McGraw-Hill Companies, Inc; 2007: 507.

41. Tremblay GB, Giguère V. Coregulators of estrogen receptor action. *Crit Rev Eukaryot Gene Expr.* 2002; 12(1):1-22.

42. Mosselman S, Polman J, Dijkema R. ER beta: Identification and Characterization of a Novel Human Estrogen Receptor. *FEBS Lett.* 1996; 392(1):49-53.

43. Arts J, Kuiper GG, Janssen JM, Gustafsson JA, Löwik CW, Pols HA, van Leewuwen JP. Differential expression of estrogen receptors alpha and beta mRNA during differentiation of human osteoblast SV-HFO cells. *Endocrinology.* 1997; 138(11):5067-70.

44. Nilsson S, Gustafsson JA. Estrogen receptor transcription and transactivation: Basic aspects of estrogen action. *Breast Cancer Res.* 2000; 2(5): 360-366.

45. Miller VM, Duckles SP. Vascular Actions of Estrogen: Functional Implications. *Pharmacol Rev.* 2008; 60(20): 210-241.

46. Doherty TM, AsotraK, Fitzpatrick LA, et al. Calcification in atherosclerosis: Bone biology and chronic inflammation at the arterial crossroads. *Proc Natl Acad Sci USA*. 2003; 100(20):11201-6

47. Vandershueren D, Gaytant J, Boonen S, Venken K. Androgens and Bone. *Curr Opin Endocrinol Diabetes Obes*. 2008; 15(3):250-4.

48. Gennari L, Merlotti D, De Paola V, Calabrò A, Becherini L, Martini G, Nuti R. Estrogen receptor gene polymorphisms and the genetics of osteoporosis: A Huge review. *Am J Epidemiol*. 2005; 161(4):307-20.

49. Gardner DG, Shoback D. *Greenspan's Basic & Clinical Endocrinology*. 8th ed. McGraw-Hill Companies, Inc; 2007: 541.

50. Van Cromphaut SJ, Rummens K, Stockmans I, et al. Intestinal calcium transporter genes are upregulated by estrogens and the reproductive cycle through vitamin D receptor-independent mechanisms. *Bone Miner Res*. 2003; 18(10):1725-36.

51. Porterfield SP, White BA. *Endocrine Physiology*. 3rd ed. Mosby, Inc; 2007: 248.

52. Rybacztk LA, Bashaw MJ, Pathak DR, et al. Serotonergic Mediation of Estrogen-Related Physiology and Physiology. *BMC Women's Health*. 2005; 5:12. doi: 10.1186/1472-6874-5-12.

53. Tuckey RC. Progesterone synthesis by the human placenta. Placenta. 2005Apr; 26(4):273-81.

54. Sherwin BB. Estrogen and cognitive aging in women. *Trends Pharmacol Sci*. 2002; 23(11):527-34.

55. Cyr M, Calon F, Morissette M, Di Paolo T. Estrogenic modulation of brain activity: implications for schizophrenia and Parkinson's disease. *J Psychiatry*

Neurosci. 2002; 27(1): 12-27.

56. Smith CC, Vedder LC, McMahon LL. Estradiol and the relationship between dendritic spines, NR2B containing NMDA receptors, and the magnitude of long-term potentiation at hippocampal CA3-CA1 synapses. *Psychoneuroendocrinology.* 2009. http://dx.doi. org/10.1016/j.psyneuen.2009.06.003.

57. Hall JM, McDonnell DP. Coregulators in nuclear estrogen receptor action: from concept to therapeutic targeting. *Mol Interv.* 2005; 5(6):343-57.

58. Toran-Allerand CD. Minireview: A plethora of estrogen receptors in the brain: where will it end? *Endocrinology.* 2004; 145(3):1069-74.

59. McEwen BS. Invited review: Estrogens effects on the brain: multiple sites and molecular mechanisms. *J Appl Physiol.* 2001; 91(6):2785-801.

60. McCullough LD, Hurn PD. Estrogen and ischemic neuroprotection: an integrated view. *Trends Endocrinol Metab.* 2003; 14(5):228-35.

61. Azcoitia I, Doncarios LL, Garcia-Segura LM. Estrogen and brain vulnerability. *Neurotox Res.* 2002; 4(3):235-45.

62. Sherwin BB. Estrogen and Cognitive Functioning in Women. *Endocrine Reviews.* 2003; 24(2):133-151.

63. Nilsen J, Brinton RD. Impact of progestins on estrogen-induced neuroprotection: synergy by progesterone and 19-norprogesterone and antagonism by medroxyprogesterone acetate. *Endocrinology.* 2002; 143(1):205-12.

64. Brandes JL. The influence of estrogen on migraine: a systemic review. *JAMA.* 2006; 295(15):1824-30.

65. MacGregor EA, Frith A, Ellis J, Aspinall L, Hackshaw A. Incidence of migraine relative to menstrual cycle phases of rising and falling estrogen. *Neurology.* 2006; 67(12):2154-8.

66. Mikkola T, Viinikka L, Ylikorkala O. Estrogen and postmenopausal estrogen/progestin therapy: effect on endothelium-dependant prostacyclin, nitric oxide and endothelin-1 production. *Eur J Obstet Gynecol Reprod Biol.* 1998; 79(1):75-82.

67. Barton M, Meyer MR. Postmenopausal Hypertension. *Hypertension.* 2009; 54:11-18.

68. Gallagher PE, Li P, Lenhart JR, Chappell MC, Brosnihan KB. Estrogen regulation of angiotensin-converting enzyme mRNA. *Hypertension.* 1999; 33(1 Pt 2):323-8.

69. Ashraf MS, Vongpatanasin W. Estrogen and hypertension. *Curr Hypertens Rep.* 2006; 8(5):368-76.

70. Bracamonte MP, Miller VM. Vascular effects of estrogens: arterial protection versus venous thrombotic risk. *Trends Endocrinol Metab.* 2001; 12(5):204-9.

71. Bush DE, Jones CE, Bass KM, Walters GK, Bruza JM, Ouyang P. Estrogen replacement reverses endothelial dysfunction in postmenopausal women. *Am J Med.* 1998; 104(6):552-8.

72. Cid MC, Schnaper HW, Kleinman HK. Estrogens and vascular endothelium. *Ann N Y Acad Sci.* 2002; 966:143-57.

73. Savolainen-Peltonen H, Loubtchenkov M, Petrov L, Delafontaine P, Häyry P. Estrogen regulates insulin-like growth factor 1, platelet-derived growth factor A and B, and their receptors in the vascular wall. *Transplantation.* 2004; 77(1):35-42.

74. Morey AK, Razandi M, Pedram A, Hu RM, Prins BA,

Levin ER. Oestrogen and progesterone inhibit the stimulated production of endothelin-1. *Biochem J.* 1998; 330 (Pt 3):1097-105.

75.　Sator MO, Joura EA, Gruber DM, Wieser F, Jirecek S, Tschugguel W, Huber JC. The effect of hormone replacement therapy on carotid arteries: measurement with a high frequency ultrasound system. *Maturitas.* 1998; 30(1):63-8.

76.　Abedin M, Tintut Y, Demer LL. Vascular calcifications: mechanisms and ramifications. *Arterioscler Throm Vasc Biol.* 2004; 24(7):1161-70.

77.　Grohé C, Kahlert S, Löbbert K, Stimpel M, Karas RH, Vetter H, Neyses L. Cardiac myocytes and fibroblasts contain functional estrogen receptors. *FEBS Lett.* 1997; 416(1)107-12.

78.　Nussmeier NA, Marino MR, Vaughn WK. Hormone replacement therapy is associated with improved survival in women undergoing coronary artery bypass grafting. *J Thorac Cardiovasc Surg.* 2002; 124:1225-1229.

79.　Hernandez AM, Walker AM, Jick H. Use of replacement estrogens and the risk of myocardial infarction. *Epidemiology.* 1990; 1(2)128-33.

80.　Finucane FF, Madans JH, Bush TL, Wolf PH, Kleinman JC. Decreased risk of stroke among postmenopausal hormone users. Results from a national cohort. *Arch Intern Med.* 1993; 153(1):73-9.

81.　Falkeborn M, Persson, Terént A, Adami HO, Lithell H, Bergström R. Hormone replacement therapy and the risk of stroke. Follow-up of a population-based cohort in Sweden. *Arch Intern Med.* 1993; 153(10):1201-9.

82.　Yang SH, Liu R, Perez EJ, Wen Y, Stevens SM Jr,

Valencia T, Brun-Zinkernagel AM, Prokai L, Will Y, Dykens J, Koulen P, Simpkins JW. Mitochondrial localization of estrogen receptor beta. *Proc Natl Acad Sci USA.* 2004; 101(12):4130-5.

83. Psarra AM, Sekeris CE. Steroid and thyroid hormone receptors in mitochondria. *IUBMB Life.* 2008; 60(4):210-23.

84. Scheller K, Sekeris CE. The effects of steroid hormones on the transcription of genes encoding enzymes of oxidative phosphorylation. Exp Physiol. 2003 Jan; 88(1):129-40.

85. Scheller K, Seibel P, Sekeris CE. Glucocorticoid and thyroid hormone receptors in mitochondria of animal cells. *Int Rev Cytol.* 2003; 222:1-61.

86. Psarra AM, Solakidi S, Sekeris CE. The mitochondrion as a primary site of action of steroid and thyroid hormones: presence and action of steroid and thyroid hormone receptors in mitochondria of animal cells. *Mol Cell Endocrinol.* 2006; 246(1-2):21-33.

87. Veldhuis JD, Keenan DM, Bowers CY. Peripheral estrogen receptor-alpha selectivity modulates the waveform of GH secretory bursts in healthy women. *Am J Physiol Regulatory, Integrative and Comparative Physiol.* 2007; 293(4):R1514-21.

88. Leung K-C, Johannsson G, Leong GM, Ho KKY. Estrogen regulation of Growth Hormone Action. *Endocr Rev.* 2004; 25:693-721.

89. Verdier-Sévrain S, Bronté F, Gilchrest B. Biology of estrogens in skin: implications for skin aging. *Exp Dermatol.* 2006; 15: 83-94.

90. Mao A, Paharkova-Vatchkova V, Hardy J, Miller MM, Kovats S. Estrogen selectivity promotes the

differentiation of dendritic cells with characteristics of Langerhans cells. *J Immunol.* 2005; 175(8):5146-51.

91.   Grimaldi CM, Hill L, Xu X, Peeva E, Diamond B. Hormonal modulation of B cell development and repertoire selection. *Mol Immunol.* 2005; 42(7):811-20.

92.   Grimaldi CM. Sex and systemic lupus erythematosus: the role of the sex hormones estrogens and prolactin on the regulation of autoreactive B cells. *Curr Opin Rheumatol.* 2006; 18(5):456-61.

93.   Mudali S, Dobs AS, Ding J, Cauley JA, Szklo M, Golden SH. Endogenous Postmenopausal Hormones and Serum Lipids: The Atherosclerosis Risk in Communities Study. *J Clin Endocrinol Metab.* 2005; 90(2):1202-1209.

94.   Barnett JB, Woods MN, Lamon-Fava S, Schaefer EJ, McNamara JR, Spiegelman D, Hertzmark E, Goldin B, Longcope C, Gorbach SL. Plasma Lipid and Lipoprotein Levels during the Follicular and Luteal Phases of the Menstrual Cycle. *J Clin Endocrinol Metab.* 2004; 89(2):776-782.

95.   Bush TL, Barrett-Connor E, Cowen LD, Criqui MH Wallace RB, Suchindran CM, Tyroler HA, Rifkind BM. Cardiovascular mortality and noncontraceptive use of estrogen in women: results from the Lipid Research Clinics Program Follow-up Study. *Circulation.* 1987; 75(6):1102-9.

96.   Thornton MJ. Biological actions of estrogen on the skin. *Exp Dermatol.* 2002; 11(6):487-502.

97.   Verdier-Sévrain S, Bronté F, Gilchrest B. Biology of estrogen in skin: implications for skin aging. *Exp Dermatol.* 2006; 15(2):83-94.

98.   Kasperska-Zajac A, Brzoza Z, Rogala B. Sex hormones and urticaria. *J Dermatol Sci.* 2008; 52(2):79-86.

99. Young T. Menopause, Hormone Replacement Therapy, and Sleep-disordered Breathing. *Am J Respir Crit Care Med.* 2001; 163(3):597-598.

100. Brown M. Skeletal muscle and bone: effect of sex steroids and aging. Adv Physiol Edu. 2008; 32:120-126.

101. Bodó E, Kromminga A, Bíró T, Borbíró I, Gaspar E, et al. Human female hair follicles are a direct, nonclassical target for thyroid-stimulating hormone. *J Invest Dermatol.* 2009; 129(5):1126-39.

102. Porterfield SP, White BA. *Endocrine Physiology.* 3rd ed. Mosby, Inc; 2007: 282.

103. Peluso JJ. Non-genomic actions of progesterone in the normal and neoplastic mammalian ovary. *Semin Reprod Med.* 2007; 25(3):198-207.

104. Berne RM, Levy MN. Physiology. 3rd ed. Mosby Year Book, Inc; 1993: 1012.

105. Singh M. Mechanisms of progesterone-induced neuroprotection. *Ann N Y Acad Sci.* 2005; 1052:145-51.

106. Reddy DS. Role of neurosteroids in catamenial epilepsy. *Epilepsy Res.* 2004; 62(2-3):99-118.

107. Reddy DS, Rogawski MA. Neurosteroid replacement therapy for catamenial epilepsy. *Neurotherapeutics.* 2009; 6(2):392-401.

108. Stein DG. Progesterone Exerts Neuroprotective Effects After Brain Injury. *Brain Res Rev.* 2008; 57(2)386-397.

109. Gonzalez SL, Labombarda F, Deniselle MC, et al. Progesterone neuroprotection in spinal cord trauma involves up-regulation of brain-derived neurotrophic factor in motoneurons. *J Steroid Biochem Mol Biol.*

2005; 94(1-3):143-9.

110. De Nicola AF, Gonzalez SL, Labombarda F, Deniselle MC, Garay L, Guennoun R, Schumacher M. Progesterone treatment of spinal cord injury: Effects on receptors, neurotrophins, and myelination. *J Mol Neurosci.* 2006; 28(1):3-15.

111. Singh M. Progesterone-induced neuroprotection. *Endocrine.* 2006; 29(2):271-4

112. Nilsen J, Morales A, Brinton RD. Medroxyprogesterone acetate exacerbates glutamate excitotoxicity. Gynecol Endocrinol. 2006 Jul; 22(7):355-61.

113. Campagnoli C, Clavel-Chapelon F, Kaaks R, Peris C, Berrino F. Progestins and progesterone in hormone replacement therapy and the risk of breast cancer. *J Steroid Biochem Mol Biol.* 2005; 96(2): 95-108.

114. Micevych P, Sinchak K. Estradiol regulation of progesterone synthesis in the brain. *Mol Cell Endocrinol.* 2008; 290(1-2):44-50.

115. Vassilopoulou-Sellin R, Asmar L, Hortobagyi GN, Klein MJ, McNeese M, Singletary SE, Theriault RL. Estrogen replacement therapy after localized breast cancer: clinical outcome of 319 women followed prospectively. *J Clin Oncol.* 1999; 17(5):1482-7.

116. Chaffkin LM, Lucciano AA, Peluso JJ. The role of progesterone in regulating human granulosa cell proliferation and differentiation in vitro. *J Clin Endocrinol Metab.* 1993; 76(3):696-700.

117. Chaffkin LM, Lucciano AA, Peluso JJ. Progesterone as an autocrine/paracrine regulator of human granulosa cell proliferation. *J Clin Endocrinol Metab.* 1992; 75(6):1404-8.

118. Engmann L, Losel R, Wehling M, Peluso JJ. Progesterone

regulation of human granulosa/luteal cell viability by an RU486-independent mechanism. *J Clin Endocrinol Metab*. 2006; 91(12):4962-8.

119. Otsuki M, Saito H, Xu X, Sumitani S, Kouhara H, Kishimoto T, Kasayama S. Progesterone, but Not Medroxyprogesterone, Inhibits Vascular Cell Adhesion Molecule-1 Expression in Human Vascular Endothelial Cell. *Arteriosclerosis, Thrombosis, and Vascular Biology*. 2001; 21:243.

120. Ghatge RP, Jacobsen BM, Schittone SA, Horwitz KB. The progestational and androgenic properties of medroxyprogesterone acetate: gene regulatory overlap with dihydrotestosterone in breast cancer cells. *Breast Cancer Res*. 2005; 7(6):R1036-50.

121. Nilsen J, Brinton RD. Divergent impact of progesterone and medroxyprogesterone acetate (provera) on nuclear mitogen-activated protein kinase signaling. *Proc Natl Acad Sci U S A*. 2003; 100(18):10506-11.

122. Meendering JR, Torgrimson BN, Miller NP, Kaplan PF, Minson CT. Estrogen, medroxyprogesterone acetate, endothelial function, and biomarkers of cardiovascular risk in young women. *Am J Physiol Heart Circ Physiol*. 2008; 294:H1630-H1637.

123. Booth EA, Lucchesi BR. Medroxyprogesterone acetate prevents the cardioprotective and anti-inflammatory effects of 17ß-estradiol in an in vivo model of myocardial ischemia and reperfusion. *Am J Physiol Heart Circ Physiol*. 2007; 293:H1408-H1415.

124. Lamon-Fava S, Postfai B, Diffenderfer M, et al. Role of the Estrogen and Progestin in Hormonal Replacement Therapy on Apolipoprotein A-1 Kinetics in Postmenopausal Women. *Arteriosclerosis, Thrombosis, and Vascular Biology*. 2006; 26:385.

125. Thomas P. Characteristics of membrane progestin receptor alpha (mPRalpha) and progesterone membrane receptor component 1 (PGMRC1) and their roles in mediating rapid progestin actions. *Front Neuroendocrinol.* 2008; 29(2):292-312.

126. Liepa G, Sengupta A, Karsies D. Polycystic Ovary Syndrome (PCOS) and Other Androgen Excess-Related Conditions: Can Changes in Dietary Intake Make a Difference? *Nutrition in Clinical Practice.* 2008; 23(1):63-71.

127. Mueller A, Schöfl C, Dittrich R, Cupisiti S, Oppelt PG, Schild RL, Beckman MW, Häberle L. Thyroid-stimulating hormone is associated with insulin resistance independently of body mass index and age in women with polycystic ovary syndrome. *Hum Reprod.* 2009; 24(11):2924-2930. doi:10-1093/humrep/dep285.

128. Maggio M, Lauretani F, Ceda GP, et L. Association of hormonal dysregulation with metabolic syndrome in older women: data from the InCHIANTI study. *Am J Physiol Endocrinol Metab.* 2006; 292:E353-E358.

129. Chen M-J, Yang W-S, Yang J-H, Hsiao CK, Yang Y-S, Ho H-N. Low sex hormone-binding globulin is associated with low high-density lipoprotein cholesterol and metabolic syndrome in women with PCOS. *Hum Reprod.* 2006; 21(9):2266-2271.

130. Sowers MR, Matthews KA, Jannausch M, et al. Hemostatic Factors and Estrogen during the Menopausal Transition. *J Clin Endocrinol Metab.* 2005; 90:5942-5948.

131. Goldman JA, The Women's Health Initiative 2004 – Review and Critique. *MedGenMed.* 2004; 6(3):65.

132. The North American Menopause Society. WHI estrogen only arm: overall results neutral. April 2004. The

Women's Health Initiative Steering Committee. Effects of conjugated equine estrogen in postmenopausal women with hysterectomy: the Women's Health Initiative randomized control trial. *JAMA* 2004; 291:1701-1712.

133. Nichols KC, Schenkel L, Benson H. 17 beta-estradiol for postmenopausal estrogen replacement therapy. *Obstet Gynecol Surv.* 1984; 39(4):230-45.

134. Canonico M, Oger E, Plu-Bureau G, et al; for the Estrogen and Thromboembolism Risk (ESTHER) Study Group. Hormone Therapy and Venous Thromboembolism among Postmenopausal Women: Impact of the Route of Estrogen Administration and Progestogens: The ESTHER Study. *Circulation.* 2007;115: 840-845.

135. Grady D, Herrington D, Bittner V, et al; HERS Research Group. Cardiovascular disease outcomes during 6.8 years of hormone therapy: Heart and Estrogen/progestin Replacement Study follow up (HERS II). *JAMA.* 2002; 288(1):49-57.

136. Grodstein F, Manson JE, Stampfer MJ. Postmenopausal hormone use and secondary prevention of coronary events in the nurses' health study: A prospective, observational study. *Ann Intern Med.* 2001; 135(1):1-8.

137. Barrett-Connor E, Stuenkel C. Hormones and heart disease in women: Heart and Estrogen/Progestin Replacement Study in perspective. *J Clin Endocrinol Metab.* 1999; 84(6):1848-53.

138. The Writing Group for the PEPI Trial. Effects of Estrogen or Estrogen/Progestin Regimens on Heart Disease Risk Factors in Postmenopausal Women. *JAMA.* 1995; 273(3):199-208.

139. Nachtigall LE, Nachtigall RH, Nachtigall RD, Beckman EM. Estrogen replacement therapy II: a prospective study in the relationship to carcinoma and cardiovascular and

metabolic problems. *Obstet Gynecol.* 1979; 54(1):74-9.

140. Schairer C, Adami HO, Hoover R, Persson I. Cause-specific mortality in women receiving hormone replacement therapy. *Epidemiology.* 1997; 8(1):59-65.

141. Iwaski M, Otani T, Inoue M Sasazuki S, Tsugane S; Japan Public Health Center-based Prospective Study Group. Role and impact of menstrual and reproductive factors on breast cancer risk in Japan. *Eur J Cancer Prev.* 2007; 16(2):116-23.

142. Russo J. Moral R, Balogh GA, Mailo D, Russo IH. The protective role of pregnancy in breast cancer. *Breast Cancer Res.* 2005; 7(13):131-42. Epub 2005 Apr 7.

143. Corrao G, Zambon A, Conti V, et al. Menopause hormone replacement therapy and cancer risk: an Italian record linkage investigation. *Ann Oncol.* 2008; 19(1):150-5. Epub 2007 Sep 4.

144. Mustafa IA, Bland KI. Physiological Effects of Steroid Hormones and Postmenopausal Hormone Replacement on the Female Breast and Breast Cancer Risk. Annals of Surgery. 1998; 228(5):638-651.

145. Mørch LS, Løkkegaard E, Andeasen AH, Krüger-Kjaer S, Lidegaard O. Hormone therapy and ovarian cancer. *JAMA.* 2009; 302(3):298-305.

146. Eilertsen AL, Høibraaten E, Os I, Anderson TO, Sandvik L, Sandset PM. The effects of oral and transdermal hormone replacement therapy on C-reactive protein levels and other inflammatory markers in women with high risk of thrombosis. *Maturitas.* 2005; 52(2):111-8.

147. Vehkavaara S, Silveira A, Hakala-Ala-Pietilä T, et al. Effects of oral and transdermal estrogen replacement therapy on markers of coagulation, fibrinolysis, inflammation and serum lipids and lipoproteins in

postmenopausal women. *Thromb Haemost.* 2001; 85(4):619-25.

148. Vongpatanasin W, Tuncel M, Mansour Y, Arbique D, Victor RG. Transdermal estrogen replacement therapy decrease sympathetic activity in postmenopausal women. *Circulation.* 2001; 103(24):2903-8.

149. De Lignieres B, Basdevant A, Thomas G, et al. Biological effects of estradiol-17 beta in postmenopausal women: oral versus percutaneous administration. *J Clin Endocrinol Metab.* 1986; 62(3):536-41.

150. Marinka S. Post, M. Christella, L.G.D Thomassen, et al. Effect of Oral and Transdermal Estrogen Replacement Therapy on Hemostatic Variables Associated With Venous Thrombosis. *Arteriosclerosis, Thrombosis, and Vascular Biology.* 2003; 23:1116.

151. Caufriez A. Hormonal replacement therapy (HRT) in postmenopause: a reappraisal. *Ann Endocrinol (Paris).* 2007; 68(4):241-50. Epub 2007 Jul 24.

152. Løkkegaard E, Andreasen AH, Jacobsen RK, Nielsen LH, Agger H, Lidegaard Ø. Hormone therapy and risk of myocardial infarction: a national register study. *European Heart Journal.* 2008; 29(21):2660-2668.

153. Rabbani LE, Seminario NA, Sciacca RR, Chen HJ, Giardina E-GV. Oral conjugated equine estrogen increases plasma von Willebrand factor in postmenopausal women. *J Am Coll Cardiol.* 2002; 40:1991-1999.

154. Filipsson H, Johannsson G. Growth hormone replacement in adults: interactions with other pituitary hormone deficiencies and replacement therapies. *Eur J Endocrinol.* 2009; 161:S85.

155. Hong L, Colpan A, Peptan IA, Daw J, George A, Evans CA. 17-Beta estradiol enhances osteogenic and

adipogenic differentiation of human adipose-derived stromal cells. *Tissue Eng.* 2007; 13(6):1197-203.

156. Somboonporn W. Testosterone therapy for postmenopausal women: efficacy and safety. *Semin Reprod Med.* 2006; 24(2):115-24.

157. Davis SR, Moreau M, Kroll R, et al. Testosterone for Low Libido in Postmenopausal Women Not Taking Estrogen. *N Engl J Med* 2008; 359:2409-2412.

158. Allen N, Key TJ, Dossus L, et al. Endogenous sex hormones and endometrial cancer risk in women in the European Prospective Investigation into cancer and Nutrition (EPIC). *Endocr Relat Cancer.* 2008; 15(2): 485-497.

159. Schufelt CL, Braunstein GD. Safety of testosterone use in women. *Maturitas.* 2009; 63(1):63-6. Epub 2009 Feb 27.

160. Henderson GC, Dhatariya K, Ford GC, et al. Higher muscle protein synthesis in women and men across lifespan, and failure of androgen administration to amen age-related decrements. *The FASEB Journal.* 2009; 23:631-641.

161. Dorte G, Anderson M, Hagen C, et al. Evaluation of metabolic risk markers in polycystic ovary syndrome (PCOS). Adiponectin, ghrelin, leptin and body composition in hirsute PCOS patients and controls. *European Journal of Endocrinology.* 2006; 155(2): 337-345.

162. Saad F, Gooren LJ, Haider A, Yassin A. A Dose-Response Study of Testosterone on Sexual Dysfunction and features of the Metabolic Syndrome Using Testosterone Gel and Parental Testosterone Undeconoate. Journal of Andrology. 2008; 29(1).doi:10.2164/ jandrol.107.002774.

163. Porterfield SP, White BA. *Endocrine Physiology.* 3rd ed. Mosby, Inc; 2007: 204.

164. Porterfield SP, White BA. *Endocrine Physiology.* 3rd ed. Mosby, Inc; 2007: 207

165. Gruenewald DA, Matsumato AM. Testosterone supplementation therapy for older men: potential benefits and risks. *J Am Geriatr Soc.* 2003; 51(1):101-15.

166. Tivesten Å, Vandenput L, Labrie F, Karlsson MK, Ljunggren Ö, Mellström D, Ohlsson Claes. Low Serum Testosterone and Estradiol Predict Mortality in Elderly Men. *J Clin Endocrinol Metab.* 2008; 94(7):2482-2488.

167. Laughlin GA, Barrett-Connor E, Bergstrom J. Low Serum Testosterone and Mortality in Older Men. *J Clin Endocrinol Metab.* 2007; 93(1): 68-75.

168. Vermeulen A, Kaufman JM, Goemaere S, van Pottelberg I. Estradiol in elderly men. *Aging Male.* 2002; 5(2):98-102.

169. Bhasin S, Woodhouse L, Casaburi R, et al. Testosterone dose-response relationships in healthy young men. *Am J Physiol Endocrinol Metab.* 2001; 281(6): E1172-E1181.

170. Tan RS, Pu SJ. A pilot study on the effects of testosterone in hypogonadal aging male patients with Alzheimer's disease. *Aging Male.* 2003; 6(1):13-7.

171. Stillman MJ. Testosterone replacement therapy for treatment refractory cluster headache. *Headache.* 2006; 46(6):925-33.

172. Rinnab L, Gust K, Hautmann RE, Küfer R. Testosterone replacement therapy and prostate cancer. The current position 67 years after the Huggins myth. Urology A. 2009; 48(5):516-22.

173. Wang C, Swerdloff RS, Iranmanesh A, et al. *J Clin Endocrinol Metab.* 2000; 85(8):2839-53.

174. Wang C, Alexander G, Berman N, et al. Testosterone replacement therapy improves mood in hypogonadal men - a clinical research center study. *J Clin Endocrinol Metab.* 1996; 81(10):3578-83.

175. Webb CM, McNeil JG, Hayward CS, de Zeigler D, Collins P. Effects of testosterone on coronary vasomotor regulation in men with coronary heart disease. *Circulation.*1999; 100(16):1690-6.

176. Register TC, Adams MR. Coronary artery and cultured aortic smooth muscle cells express mRNA for both the classical estrogen receptor and the newly described estrogen receptor beta. *J Steroid Biochem Mol Biol.* 1998; 64(3-4):187-91.

177. Yeap BB, Hyde Z, Almeida OP, et al. Lower Testosterone Levels Predict Incident Stroke and Transient Ischemic Attack in Older Men. J Clin Endocrinol Metab. 2008; 94(7):2353-2359.

178. Bondanelli M, Ambrosio MR, Margutti A, Franceschetti P, Zatelli MC, degli Urberti EC. Activation of the somatotropic axis by testosterone in adult men: evidence for a role of hypothalamic growth hormone-releasing hormone. *Neuroendocrinology.* 2003; 77(6):380-7.

179. Veldhuis JD, Keenan DM, Bailey JN, et al. Estradiol Supplementation in Postmenopausal Women Attenuates Suppression of Pulsatile Growth Hormone Secretion by Recombinant Human Insulin-like Growth Factor Type I. J Clin Endocrinol Metab. 2008; 93(11): 4471-4478.

180. Kupelian V, Hayes FJ, Link CL, Rosen R, McKinlay JB. Inverse Association of Testosterone and the Metabolic Syndrome in Men is Consistent across Race and Ethnic Groups. *J Endocrinol Metab.* 2008; 93(9):3403-3410.

181. Tsai EC, Matsumoto AM, Fugimoto WY, Boyko EJ. Association of bioavailable, free, and total testosterone with insulin resistance: influence of sex hormone-binding globulin and body fat. *Diabetes Care.* 2004; 27(4):861-8.

182. Page ST, Herbst KL, Amory JK Coviello AD, Anawalt BD, Matsumoto AM, Bremner WJ. Testosterone Administration Suppresses Adiponectin Levels in Men. *Journal of Andrology.* Jan/Feb 2005; 26(1):85-92.

183. Zgliczynski S, Ossowski M, Slowinska-Srzednicka J, et al. Effect of testosterone replacement therapy on lipids and lipoproteins in hypogonadal and elderly men. *Atherosclerosis.* 1996; 121(1):35-43.

184. Tengstrand B, Carlström K, Hafström I. Bioavailable testosterone in men with rheumatoid arthritis-high frequency of hypogonadism. Rheumatology (Oxford). 2002; 41(3):285-9.

185. Bischoff-Ferrari HA, Orav EJ, Dawson-Hughes B. Additive benefit of higher testosterone levels and vitamin D plus calcium supplementation in regard to fall reduction among older men and women. *Osteoporosis Int.* 2008; 19(9): 1307-1314.

186. Snyder PJ, Peachey H, Hannoush P, et al. Effect of Testosterone Treatment on Body Composition and Muscle Strength in Men Over 65 Years of Age. *J Clin Endocrinol Metab.* 1999; 84(8):2647-2653.

187. Katznelson L, Robinson MW, Coyle CL, Lee H, Farrell CE. Effects of modest testosterone supplementation and exercise for 12 weeks on body composition and quality of life in elderly men. *European Journal of Endocrinology.* 2006; 155(6):867-875.

188. Saad Farid, Yassin A. Testosterone and Erectile Dysfunction. *Journal of Andrology.* 2008; 29(6).

doi:10.2164/jandrol.107.004630.

189. Traish AM, Guay A, Feeley R, Saad F. The Dark Side of Testosterone Deficiency: I. Metabolic Syndrome and Erectile Dysfunction. *J Androl.* 2009; 30(1).doi:10.2164/jandrol.108.005215.

190. Seftel AD, Mack RJ, Secrest AR, Smith TM. Restorative increases in serum testosterone levels are significantly correlated to improvements in sexual functioning. *J Androl.* 2004; 25(6):963-72.

191. Mommers E, Kersemaekers WM, Elliesen J, et al. M. Male Hormonal Contraception: A Double-Blind, Placebo-Controlled Study. *J Clin Endocrinol Metab.* 2008; 93(7):2572-2580.

192. Wespes E, Schulman CC. Male andropause: myth, reality, and treatment. *Int J Impot Res.* 2002; 14 Suppl 1:S98-8.

193. Flyckt RL, Liu J, Frasure H, Wekselman K, Buch A, Kingsberg SA. Comparison of salivary versus serum testosterone levels in postmenopausal women receiving transdermal testosterone supplementation versus placebo. *Menopause.* 2009; 16:680.

194. Wood P. Salivary steroid assays - research or routine? Ann Clin Biochem. 2009; 46(Pt 3):183-96.

195. Gooren LJ. Advances in testosterone replacement therapy. *Front Horm Res.* 2009; 37:32-51.

196. Meikle AW, Arver S, Dobs AS, et al. Prostate size in hypogonadal men treated with a nonscrotal permeation-enhanced testosterone transdermal system. *Urology.* 1997; 49(2):191-6.

197. Coward RM, Simhan J, Carson CC. Prostate-specific antigen changes and prostate cancer in hypogonadal men treated with testosterone replacement therapy. *BJU.*

2009; 103(9):1179-83.

198. Morris MJ, Huang D, Kelly WK, et al. Phase 1 Trial of High-Dose Exogenous Testosterone in Patients with Castration-Resistant Metastatic Prostate Cancer. *Eur Urol.* 2009; 56(2):237-44.

199. Porterfield SP, White BA. *Endocrine Physiology.* 3rd ed. Mosby, Inc; 2007: 180

200. Porterfield SP, White BA. *Endocrine Physiology.* 3rd ed. Mosby, Inc; 2007: 178-179.

201. Gardner DG, Shoback D. *Greenspan's Basic & Clinical Endocrinology.* 8th ed. McGraw-Hill Companies, Inc; 2007: 540.

202. Zang H, Davis SR. Androgen replacement therapy in androgen-deficient women with hypopituitarism. *Drugs.* 2008; 68(15):2085-93.

203. Hahner S, Allolio B. Therapeutic management of adrenal insufficiency. *Best Pract Res Clin Endocrinol Metab.* 2009; 23(2):167-79.

204. Srinivasan M, Irving BA, Dhatariya K, Klaus KA, Hartman SJ, McConnell JP, Nair KS. Effect of dehydroepiandrosterone replacement on lipoprotein profile in hypoadrenal women. *J Clin Endocrinol Metab.* 2009; 94(3):761-4. Epub 2008 Dec 9.

205. Gardner DG, Shoback D. *Greenspan's Basic & Clinical Endocrinology.* 8th ed. McGraw-Hill Companies, Inc; 2007: 351.

206. Jenkinson DM, Harbert AJ. Supplements and sports. *Am Fam Physician.* 2008; 78(9):1039-46.

207. Furay AR, Bruestle AE, Herman JP. The Role of the Forebrain Glucocorticoid Receptors in Acute and Chronic Stress. *Endocrinology.* 2008; 149(11):5482-

5490.

208. Walker BR. Glucocorticoids and Cardiovascular Disease. *Eur J Endocrinol.* 2007; 157(5):545-559.

209. Porterfield SP, White BA. *Endocrine Physiology.* 3rd ed. Mosby, Inc; 2007: 186-187.

210. Okuneva V, Zhvania M, Japaridze N, Gelazonia L, Lordkipanidze T. Stress-system: corticotropin-releasing hormone and catecholamines (review). *Georgian Med News.* 2009; (172-173):65-9.

211. van Hoek I, Daminet S. Interactions between thyroid and kidney function in pathological conditions of these organ systems: a review. *Gen Comp Endocrinol.* 2009; 160(3):205-15.

212. Iglesias P, Díez JJ. Thyroid dysfunction and kidney disease. *Eur J Endocrinol.* 2009; 160(4):503-15.

213. Portman MA. Thyroid hormone regulation of heart metabolism. *Thyroid.* 2008; 18(2):217-25.

214. Danzi S, Klein I. Thyroid hormone regulated cardiac gene expression and cardiovascular disease. *Thyroid.* 2002; 12(6):467-72.

215. Oetting A, Yen PM. New insight into thyroid hormone action. *Best Pract Res Clin Endocrinol Metab.* 2007; 21(2):193-208.

216. Malik R, Hodgson H. The relationship between the thyroid gland and the liver. *QJM.* 2002; 95(9):559-69.

217. O'Brian T, Dinneen SF, O'Brian PC, Palumbo PJ. Hyperlipidemia in patients with primary and secondary hypothyroidism. *N Engl J Med.* 1993; 328:1069-1075.

218. Tan ZS, Vasan RS. Thyroid function and Alzheimer's disease. *J Alzheimer's Dis.* 2009; 16(3):503-7.

219. Goumidi L, Flamant F, Lendon C, et al. Study of thyroid hormone receptor alpha gene polymorphisms on Alzheimer's disease. *Neurobiol Aging.* 2009; 6.doi:10.1016/j.neurobiolaging.2009.04.007.

220. Kelly T, Lieberman DZ. The use of triiodothyronine as an agent in treatment-resistant bipolar II and bipolar disorders NOS. *Affect Disord.* 2009; 116(3):222-6

221. Nunez J, Celi FS, Ng L, Forrest D. Multigenic control of thyroid hormone functions in the nervous system. *Mol Cell Endocrinol.* 2008; 287(1-2):1-12.

222. Anderson GW. Thyroid hormone and cerebellar development. *Cerebellum.* 2008; 7(1):60-74.

223. Rosenfeld RS. The future of research into growth hormone responsiveness. *Horm Res.* 2009; 71 Suppl 2:71-4.

224. Sirotkin A, Ovcharenko D, Mlyncek M. Identification of protein kinases that control ovarian hormone release by selective siRNAs. J Mol Endocrinol. 2009 Aug 27.

225. Woodhouse LJ, Mukherjee A, Shalet SM, Ezzat S. The influence of growth hormone status on physical impairments, functional limitations, and health-related quality of life in adults. *Endocr Rev.* 2006; 27(3):287-317.

226. Rudman D, Feller AG, Nagrai HS, et al. Effects of human growth hormone in men over 60 years old. *N Engl J Med.* 1990; 323(1):1-6.

227. Muniyappa R, Sorkin JD, Veldhuis JD, et al. Long-term testosterone supplementation augments overnight growth hormone secretion in healthy older men. *Am J Physiol Endocrinol Metab.* 2007; 293(3):E769-75.

228. Sattler FR, Castaneda-Sceppa C, Binder EF, et al. Testosterone and Growth Hormone Improve Body

Composition and Muscle performance in Older Men. *J Clin Endocrinol Metab.* 1991-2001; 94(6):2008-2338.

229. Vermeulen A, Goemaere S, Kaufman JM. Testosterone, body composition and aging. *J Endocrinol Invest.* 1999; 22(5Suppl):110-6.

230. Vermeulen A. Aging, hormones, body composition, metabolic effects. *World J Urol.* 2002; 20(1):23-7.

231. Rodríguez-Arnao J, Jabbar A, Fulcher K, Besser GM, Ross RJ. Effects of growth hormone replacement on physical performance and body composition in GH deficient adults. *Clin Endocrinol (Oxf).* 1999; 51(1):53-60.

232. Kato K, Suzuki M, Kanno H, et al. Distinct role of growth hormone on epilepsy progression in a model of temporal lobe epilepsy. *Neurochem.* 2009; 110(2):509-19

233. Chrisoulidou A, Kousta E, Beshyah SA, Robinson S, Johnston DG. How much, and by what mechanisms, does growth hormone replacement improve the quality of life in GH-deficient adults? *Baillieres Clin Endocrinol Metab.* 1998;12(2):261-79.

234. Wallymahmud ME, Foy P, Shaw D, Hutcheon R, Edwards RH, MacFarlane IA. Quality of life, body composition and muscle strength in adult growth hormone deficiency: the influence of growth hormone replacement therapy for up to 3 years. *Clin Endocrinol (Oxf).* 1997; 47(4):439-46.

235. Thomas J, Monson J. Adult growth hormone deficiency throughout lifetime. *Eur J Endocrinol.* 2009; 161:S97.

236. Ma QL, Yang TL, Yin JY, et al. Role of insulin like growth factor-1 (IGF-1) in regulating cell cycle progression. *Biochem Biophys Res Commun.* 2009;doi:10.1016/j.

bbrc.2009.08.114.

237. Kokoszko A, Lewiński A, Karbownik-Lewińska M. The role of growth hormone and insulin-like growth factor 1 in oxidative processes. *Endokrynol Pol.* 2008; 59(6):496-501.

238. Cuatrecasas G. Fibromyalgia syndromes: could growth hormone therapy be beneficial? *Pediatr Endocrinol Rev.* 2009; 6 Suppl 4.

239. Sanders EJ, Parker E, Harvey S. Endogenous growth hormone in human retinal ganglion cells correlates with cell survival. *Mol Vis.* 2009; 15:920-6.

240. Morrhaye G, Kermani H, Legros JJ, et al. Impact of growth hormone (GH) replacement upon thymus function in adult patients. *PLos One.* 2009; 4(5):e5668.

241. Veldhuis JD, Bowers CY. Determinants of GH-releasing hormone and GH-releasing peptide synergy in men. *Am J Physiol Endocrinol Metab.* 2009; 296:E1085-1092.

242. Weltman A, Weltman JY, Hartman ML, Abbott RD, Rogol AD, Evans WS, Veldhuis JD. Relationship between age, percentage body fat, fitness, and 24-hour growth hormone release in healthy young adults: effects of gender. *J Clin Endocrinol Metab.* 1994; 78:543-548.

243. Veldhuis JD, Hudson SB, Erickson D, Bailey JN, Reynolds GA, Bowers CY. Relative effects of estrogen, age and visceral fat on pulsatile growth hormone secretion in healthy women. *Am J Physiol Endocrinol Metab.* 2009; 297(2):E367-74.

244. Veldhuis JD, Hudson SA, Bailey, Erickson D. Regulation of basal, pulsatile, and entropic (patterned) modes of GH secretion in putatively low-somatostatin milieu in women. *Am J Physiol Endocrinol Metab.* 2009; 297(2):E483-9.

245. Rosenfeld RG, Hwa V. The growth hormone cascade and its role in mammalian growth. *Horm Res*. 2009; 71 Suppl 2:36-40.

246. Spiliotis BE, Alexandrides TK, Karystianos C, et al. The insulin-like growth factor (IGF-1) generation test as an indicator of growth hormone status. *Hormones (Athens)*. 2009; 8(2):117-28.

247. Lacey JV Jr, Mink PJ, Lubin JH, et al. Menopausal hormone replacement therapy and the risk for ovarian cancer. *JAMA*. 2002; 288(3):334-41.

248. Bright GM, Mendoza JR, Rosenfeld RG. Recombinant human insulin-like growth factor-1: ready for primetime. *Endocrinol Metab Clin North Am*. 2009; 38(3) 625-38.

249. Walvoord EC, de la Peña A, Park S, et al. Inhaled growth hormone (GH) compared with subcutaneous GH in children with GH deficiency: pharmacokinetics, pharmacodynamics, and safety. *J Clin Endocrinol Metab*.2009; 94(6):2052-9.

250. Vieth R. Why "Vitamin D" is not a hormone, and not a synonym for 1,25-dihydroxy-vitamin D, its analogs or deltanoids. *Journal of Steroid Biochemistry & Molecular Biology*. 2004; 89-90:571-573.

251. Holick MF. Vitamin D: A millennium perspective. *Journal of Cellular Biochemistry*. 2002; 88(2):296-307.

252. Kriebitzsch C, Verlindin L, Esleen G, Tan BK, Van Camp M, Bouillon R, Verstuyf A. The impact of 1,25(OH)2D3 and its structural analogs on gene expression in cancer cells – a microarray approach. *Anticancer Res*. 2009; 29(9):3471-83.

253. Ambroszkiewicz J, Klemarczyk W, Gajewska J, et al. [Effect of vitamin D supplementation on serum

25-hydroxyvitamin D and bone turnover markers concentrations in vegetarian children]. *Med Wieku Rozwoj.* 2009; 13(1):34-9.

254. Camacho PM, Dayal AS, Diaz JL, et al. Prevalence of secondary causes of bone loss among breast cancer patients with osteopenia and osteoporosis. *J Clin Oncol.* 2008; 20;26(33):5380-5

255. Holick MF. Vitamin D: importance in the prevention of cancers, type 1 diabetes, heart disease, and osteoporosis. *Am J Clin Nutr.* 2004; 79(3):362-71.

256. Lu L, Yu Z, Pan A, et al. 25-Hydroxyvitamin D Concentration and Metabolic Syndrome Among Middle-Aged and Elderly Chinese Individuals. *Diabetes Care.* 2009; 32(7):1278-1283.

257. Oh J, Weng S, Felton SK, et al. 1,25(OH)2 Vitamin D Inhibits Foam Cell Formation and Suppresses Macrophage Cholesterol Uptake in Patients With Type 2 Diabetes Mellitus. *Circulation.* 2009.doi:101161/circulationaha.109856070.

258. Lind L, Hänni A, Lithell H, Hvarfner A, Sörensen OH, Ljunghall S. Vitamin D is related to blood pressure and other cardiovascular risk factors in middle-aged men. *Am J Hypertens.* 1995; 8(9):894-901.

259. Grimes DS, Hindle E, Dyer T. Sunlight, cholesterol and coronary heart disease. *QJM.* 1996; 89(8):579-89.

260. Cross HS, Nittke T, Peterlik M. Modulation of vitamin D synthesis and catabolism in colorectal mucosa: a new target for cancer prevention. *Anticancer Res.* 2009; 29(9):3705-12.

261. Peterlik M, Grant WB, Cross HS. Calcium, vitamin D and cancer. *Anticancer Res.* 2009; 29(9):3687-98.

262. Ingraham BA, Bragdon B, Nohe A. molecular basis for

the potential of vitamin D to prevent cancer. *Current Medical Research and Opinion*. 2008; 24(1):139-149.

263. Crew KD, Shane E, Cremers S, McMahon DJ, Irani D, Hershman DL. High prevalence of vitamin D deficiency despite supplementation in premenopausal women with breast cancer undergoing adjuvant chemotherapy. *J Clin Oncol.* 2009; 27(13):2151-6.

264. Crew KD, Gammon MD, Steck SE, et al. Association between plasma 25-hydroxyvitamon D and breast cancer risk. *Cancer Prev Res (Phila Pa).* 2009; 2(6):598-604.

265. Goodwin PJ, Ennis M, Prichard KI, Koo J, Hood N. Prognostic effects of 25-hydroxyvitamin D levels in early breast cancer. *J Clin Oncol.* 2009; 27(23):3757-63.

266. Nürnberg B, Gräber S, Gärtner B, Geisel J, Pföhler C, Schaddendorf D, Tilgen W, Reichrath J. Reduced serum 25-hydroxyvitamin D levels in stage IV melanoma patients. *Anticancer Res.* 2009; 29(9):3669-74.

267. Freedman DM, Looker AC, Chang SC, Graubard BI. Prospective study of serum Vitamin D and cancer mortality in the United States. *J Natl Cancer Inst.* 2007; 99(21):1594-602.

268. Krishnan AV, Peehl DM, Feldman D. The role of vitamin D in prostate cancer. *Recent Results Cancer Res.* 2003; 164:205-21.

269. Chen TC, Wang L, Whitlatch LW, Flanagan JN, Holick MF. Prostatic 25-hydroxyvitamin D-1α-hydroxylase and its implications in prostate cancer. *Journal of Cellular Biochemistry.* 2002; 88(2):315-322.

270. Lu LJ, Zha DJ, Xue T, Qiu JH. [Inhibitory effects of 1,25(OH)2D3 on proliferation of human laryngeal carcinoma cells and potential mechanisms.] *Ai Zheng.*

2009; 28(7):691-4.

271. Khan QJ, Reddy PS, Kimler BF, Sharma P, Baxa SE, O'Dea AP, Klemp JR, Fabian CJ. Effect of vitamin D supplementation on serum 25-hydroxy vitamin D levels, joint pain, and fatigue in women starting adjuvant letrozole treatment for breast cancer. *Breast Cancer Res Treat.* 2009; 119(1):111-8.

272. Al-Said YA, Al-Rached HS, Al-Qahtani HA, Jan MM. severe proximal myopathy with remarkable recovery after vitamin D treatment. *Can J Neurol Sci.* 2009; 36(3):336-9.

273. van Etten E, Mathieu C. Immunoregulation by 1,25-dihydroxyvitamin D3: Basic concepts. *Journal of Steroid Biochemistry and Molecular Biology.* 2005; 97(1-2):93-101.

274. Cannell JJ, Vieth R, Umhau JC, et al. Epidemic influenza and Vitamin D. *Epidemiol Infect.* 2006; 134(6)1129-40.

275. Shipowick CD, Moore CB, Corbett C, Bindler R. Vitamin D and depressive symptoms in women during the winter: a pilot study. *Appl Nurs Res.* 2009; 22(3):221-5.

276. Gloth FM 3rd, Alam W, Hollis B. Vitamin D vs broad spectrum phototherapy in the treatment of seasonal affective disorder. *J Nutr Health Aging.* 1999; 3(1):5-7.

277. Eloranta JJ, Hiller C, Hausler S, Stieger B, Kullak-Ublick GA. Vitamin D3 and its Nuclear Receptor Increases the Expression and Activity of the Human Proton-Coupled Folate Transporter. *Mol Pharmacol.* 2009; 76(5):1062-1071.

278. Silverthorn DU. *Human Physiology: an integrated approach.* 4th ed. San Francisco, CA. Pearson Education.

Benjamin Cummings. 2007: 237.

279. Verster GC. Melatonin and its agonists, circadian rhythms and psychiatry. *Afr J Psychiatry (Johannesbg).* 2009; 12(1):42-6.

280. Azorin JM, Kaladjian A. [Depression and circadian rhythm]. *Encephale.* 2009; 35 Suppl 2:S68-71.

281. Galli-Carminati G, Deriaz N, Bertschy G. Melatonin in treatment of chronic sleep disorders in adults with autism: a retrospective study. *Swiss Med Wkly.* 2009; 139(19-20):293-6.

282. Dominguez-Rodriguez A, Abreu-Gonzalez P, Reiter RJ. Clinical aspects of melatonin in the acute coronary syndrome. *Curr Vasc Pharmacol.* 2009; 7(3):367-73.

283. Zmijewski MA, Sweatman TW, Slominski AT. The melatonin-producing system is fully functional in retinal pigment epithelium (ARPE-19). *Mol Cell Endocrinol.* 2009; 307(1-2):211-6.

284. Huang JY, Hong YT, Chuang JI. Fibroblast growth factor 9 prevents MPP+-induced death of dopaminergic neurons and is involved in melatonin neuroprotection in vivo and in vitro. *J Neurochem.* 2009; 109(5):1400-12.

285. Rakhimmova OIu. [Melatonin and its role in gastrointestinal pathology]. *Klin Med (Mosk).* 2009; 87(3):11-8.

286. Cöl C, Dinler K, Hasdemir AO, Bugdayci G. The effect of intraperitoneal injection of melatonin on serum amylase levels in acute pancreatitis. *JOP.* 2009; 10(3):306-9.

287. Singh M. Progestins and neuroprotection: are all progestins created equal? *Minerva Endocrinol.* 2007; 32(2):95-102.

288. Mohr SB, Garland CF, Gorham ED, Grant WB, Garland

FC. Relationship between low ultraviolet B irradiance and higher breast cancer risk in 107 countries. *Breast J.* 2008; 14(3):255-60.

289. Writing Group for the Women's Health Initiative Investigators. Risks and Benefits of Estrogen plus Progestin in Healthy Postmenopausal Women. *JAMA.* 2002; 288:321-333

290. Heldring N, Pike A, Anderson S, et al. Estrogen receptors: how do they signal and what are their targets. *Physiol Rev.* 2007; 87(3):905-31

291. Stirone C, Duckles SP, Krause DN, Procaccio V. Estrogen increases mitochondrial efficiency and reduces oxidative stress in cerebral blood vessels. *Mol Pharmacol.* 2005; 68(4)956-65.

292. Karas RH, Patterson BL, Mendelsohn ME. Human vascular smooth muscle cells contain functional estrogen receptor. *Circulation.* 1994; 89(5):1943-50.

293. Van Beek N, Bodó E, Kromminga A, et al. Thyroid hormones directly alter human hair follicle functions: anagen prolongation and stimulation of both hair matrix keratinocyte proliferation and hair pigmentation. *J Clin Endocrinol Metab.* 2008; 93(11):4381-8.

294. Chang-Claude J, Andrieu N, Rookus M, et al. Epidemiological Study of Familial Breast Cancer (EMBRACE): Gene Etude Prospective Sein Ovaire (GENESPO): Genen Omgeving studies van de werkgroep Hereditiair Borstkanker Onderzoek Nederland (GEO-HEBON); International BRCA1/2 Carrier Cohort Study (IBCCS) Collaborators group: Age at menarche and menopause and breast cancer risk in the international BRCA1/2 Carrier Cohort Study. *Cancer Epidemiol Biomarkers Prev.* 2007; 16(4):740-6.

295. Zerr-Fouineau M, Chataigneau M, Blot C, Schini-

Kerth VB. Progestins overcome inhibition of platelet aggregation by endothelial cells by down-regulating endothelial NO synthase via glucocorticoid receptors. *Faseb J.* 2007; 21:265-273.

296. Mahmud K. Keeping aBreast, ways to STOP Breast Cancer. AuthorHouse. 2005

297. Llewellyn DJ, Langa KM, Lang IA. Serum 25-hydroxyvitamin D concentration and cognitive impairment. *J Geriatr Psychiatry Neurol.* 2009; 22(3):188-95.

298. Okobia MN, Bunker CH. Epidemiological risk factors for breast cancer – a review. *Niger J Clin Pract.* 2005; 8(9):35-42.

299. Qui J, Bosch MA, Tobias SC, et al. Rapid Signaling of Estrogen in Hypothalamic Neurons Involves a Novel G-Protein-Coupled Estrogen Receptor that Activates Protein Kinase C. *J Neurosci.* 2003; 23(29):9529-9540.

300. Gavrilova –Jordan LP, Price TM. Actions of steroids in mitochondria. *Semin Reprod Med.* 2007; 25(3):154-64.

301. Surya S, Horowitz JF, Goldenberg N, Sakharova A, Harber M, Cornford AS, Symons K, Barkan AL. The pattern of growth hormone delivery to peripheral tissues determines insulin-like growth factor-1 and lipolytic responses in obese patients. *J Clin Endocrinol Metab.* 2009; 94(8):2828-34.

302. Jankowski CM, Gonzansky WS, Kittelson JM, Van Pelt RE, Schwartz RS, Kohrt WM. Increases in bone mineral density in response to oral dehydroepiandrosterone replacement in older adults appear to be mediated by serum estrogens. *J Clin Endocrinol Metab.* 2008; 93(12):4767-73.